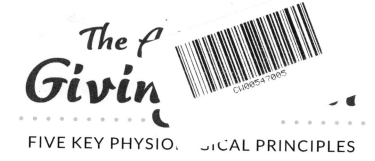

# The Art of
# Giving Birth

## FIVE KEY PHYSIOLOGICAL PRINCIPLES

*Sallyann Beresford*

DANDELION BOOKS

ISBN 978-1-8382295-1-1

First edition: October 2022

*Illustrations by Darcy Beresford*
*Cover and interior design and layout by Tessa Avila*
*Index by Tessa Avila*

10  9  8  7  6  5  4  3  2  1

Printed in the UK

*For my wonderful children —*
*Joseph, Lauren, Caitlin and Darcy*

I love you with all my heart and hope that one day
the births of your children will be as magical
as mine were with each of you.

Best wishes for
a beautiful birth

Much love

Sallyann
X X

# Contents

# Introduction

*Having a great birth isn't about luck.*

There is much to learn about having a baby, so it's no wonder Mother Nature gave us plenty of time to prepare. From the moment you became pregnant, I have no doubt you've discovered there is a wealth of information available from a wide variety of different sources. Whilst your research is probably not 100% focussed on the birth process alone, I believe that the more you can do in preparation for this life-changing event, the better. As you learn about all of your options, one philosophy regarding the way you want to give birth will most likely begin to stand out above all others. If, after your research, you think that having your baby with minimal interventions is something you are keen to explore further, then this book is for you. Its aim is to help you uncover the secrets to achieving a physiological birth. Throughout the following chapters, you will learn my five key principles and be able to decide which elements you want to take forward in preparation for your journey. Even if this isn't your goal, you can still learn ways to take ownership of your birth and help yourself to achieve a positive experience, simply by discovering more about what your body requires during labour in order to work effectively. By learning and implementing the five key physiological principles I have put together, you will be expanding your knowledge and deepening the confidence you have in your body's ability to birth in a way that should be easily achieved by the vast majority of women, but sadly is only experienced by few. This is mainly because modern maternity services follow a medicalised model of care, where a woman's body is somehow seen as an inferior product that needs drugs and devices to help it function. With interventions on the rise, most doctors and midwives are simply not seeing birth in its true form, and as such, have developed a deep lack of understanding and trust in the way the body works. Because these care providers often undermine the process with their behaviour and expectations, it has become virtually impossible for a woman to be left alone undisturbed, unless she already knows how to trust her own body and advocate for herself. Of course, planning a physiological birth isn't about avoiding good quality, safe care. It's about honouring your body's ability to give birth to your baby. When the body is left to function physiologically—in the absence of a genuine medical concern—it can be much easier for both you and your caregiver to recognise progress and feel confident that everything is going well. If it is not, and a reason to intervene arises, you can then access closer monitoring or any medical help that you or your baby need, just like you would in any other medical situation. By choosing a physiological birth, you are not ruling out receiving support; you are simply learning to trust your instincts more deeply, thereby giving you the confidence to relax and tune into your body. When the body is left alone, it works more efficiently. This undeniably leads to a much safer experience for both you and your baby.

Whether you are pregnant for the first time, or have given birth before, my hope is that you will research all of your options and come to appreciate the benefits of giving birth without medical assistance. This can be easy to achieve, when you deepen your knowledge of physiological birth and understand how to maximise your chances of having one. Throughout the book I will encourage you to identify and eliminate any doubts or fears that might get in your way, and erase any limiting beliefs that may be lying dormant inside your subconscious mind. These doubts—and those of other people—have the potential to rise up and sabotage your plans. The best way to align both your mind and your body on the day, is to ensure that not only will you 'know' your body was designed to give birth, but you will also truly believe that you 'deserve' to have a beautiful experience. In addition, as a doula and antenatal teacher for over 20 years, I am passionate about educating not only you, but also your birth partner. I want to ensure that you both feel confident in your individual roles and that whoever you choose to be with you understands and respects your preferences. That you are *both* clear about, and trust, in any decisions you are making when planning and preparing for your physiological birth. Even though you are the one going through it, the person supporting you needs to be aware of how much their presence is going to matter to you, and what you specifically need from them. Without the right support you are better off with no support—because it takes only one person who is not on board with your physiological needs to set your labour back by many hours. For this reason, there are several tools that I have put together which you can use during pregnancy to help you and your birth partner get really clear on what you want to achieve. So, by reading this book, you will begin to know who the right advocate is for you, and you can prepare them well in advance. You may even consider hiring a doula to join you and support both you and your partner. Lastly, I have a whole chapter on putting together a birth plan (see Chapter 7) so that you, your birth partner, and your care providers have a clear picture of all your preferences. This will help you to feel really well supported throughout the remainder of your pregnancy, and confident that you can easily advocate for yourselves, if any challenges come your way.

This book's aim is not to educate you to the same extent as a full antenatal course. It's intention is to take you from where you are now with your knowledge, and elevate it to the next level. I want to give you some new tools and boost your confidence, in order to support you in achieving your dream birth. I recommend you do some research into all your options locally, so that you know what locations are more likely to support your preferences. Also, where possible, consider having your baby at home or in a midwife-led unit (MLU) as opposed to a hospital, where you are more likely to experience medical intervention. For this purpose, throughout the book I will be referring to 'Plan A' as a physiological birth. This is the birth experience I am going to assume you are hoping for after learning more about my five key physiological principles. When I speak of 'Plan B,' I am referring to a managed vaginal birth. This is the birth experience you may switch to if at any time your Plan A birth shows itself to need additional support. At this point, you can change direction and make the decision to accept more intervention if it is genuinely required. And finally, 'Plan C' refers to a caesarean section, which I am choosing to call abdominal birth. Some babies have to be born via surgery despite your plan to give birth physiologically. If Plan B or C become your reality, you can still have a wonderful, positive experience, as long as you are feeling well supported and in control. My five key principles will prepare you to advocate for yourselves in any situation, because you will know how to make well informed decisions at any time. Birth trauma can occur when you feel unsafe and are coerced into making decisions that you don't fully understand. For this reason, it's really important to know how to remain in charge of 'all' the decisions you make, and how to find your voice if necessary. This ensures that any interventions you agree to lead to a positive and empowered experience, rather than a traumatic one.

The primary biological role of human beings is to survive and procreate—to conceive, grow, birth and feed another human being in order to keep our species alive. It's important to understand how the body was made to give birth, and to recognise that nature's plan was that this process would happen undisturbed. Giving birth physiologically is about learning to trust in the body, to believe in the power you have within you and to feel supported and safe whilst doing so. Any doubts, no matter how small, should be resolved with the knowledge and information you gain from within these chapters. By the end, you will have a wide range of tools that can influence the direction your birth takes, simply by enabling you to remain in control of your options at all times.

You will only have this particular pregnancy and birth journey once, so take ownership and make it an incredible, empowering experience. I want you to come away from your birth feeling that your body and your wishes were respected, that you understood every element of what your instincts were telling you, and that you kept control at all times of any decisions that needed to be made. The more confident you feel in the process, the easier you will find it to fully trust yourself, leading to a safer and more satisfying experience. Because a healthy baby is not all that matters—you matter, too.

Always remember the hero of your birth journey is not your midwife, not a doctor, or the teacher of a class that you might attend with your partner. The hero of your birth story is you.

*Much love,*
*Sallyann*

# CHAPTER ONE
# Whose Body Is It Anyway?

*You are not allowed to not allow me.*

Pregnancy is nothing short of miraculous, but it's not a walk in the park for most women. Nausea, vomiting, sore boobs, night sweats, extreme exhaustion, itching, constipation, mood changes, breathlessness, and varicose veins are just some of the symptoms that you can expect to experience. Throughout the 10 months that you are growing a whole human, your body will provide you with your own personalised set of symptoms that are unique to you and impossible to predict in advance. The changes happening inside are numerous and can leave you feeling excited one minute and in a state of turmoil the next. There are many physical and emotional symptoms that can come as a real shock to the system—in particular worrying about how your body will look, anxiety around giving birth, relationship changes, becoming a mother, and much more. As the months pass and the baby grows bigger, your body becomes flooded with hormones that soften your bones and expand your pelvis. Your internal organs begin to move and relocate inside you as the baby takes priority. New symptoms can appear, such as heartburn, the need to pee all the time, and pelvic, back, and muscle discomfort as the uterus and surrounding ligaments stretch. It's important to highlight that this incredible transition and expansion is happening within you, without you ever needing to stop and think about it. Nature's incredibly clever design ensures that the embryo's cells grow to form all parts of the baby's body, including eyes to see, ears to hear, and brains to think. Even during the last few weeks of pregnancy miraculous events are taking place. The baby's body lays down brown adipose tissue under the skin to help maintain their body temperature and keep them warm in the early days of life, whilst at the same time, your body sends healthy microbes to the birth canal and vaginal opening in preparation for the new arrival. These 'flora and fauna' will begin to seed your baby's gut during the birth process and in the moments following, helping them to develop a strong immune system.

This miraculous work is happening unconsciously within us, and we trust and believe our body knows what to do, barely pausing to question it. When it comes to the end of pregnancy, however, it is becoming increasingly common to throw all faith in the human body's ability to complete the reproduction process out the window. The 'maternity system' you are booked with may begin offering you extra checks and scans that will undoubtedly lead to interventions. Far too many women whose pregnancies have been previously straightforward can expect their care providers to begin questioning the way their baby is growing. They may express concerns to you and recommend intervening to cut short the pregnancy, with the explanation that your body could stop working efficiently at any moment, or your placenta could 'fail.' If you have not had any serious medical concerns identified, and you have decided to give birth physiologically, there is very little that can be detected in later pregnancy that should impact the way your baby is born. Women are being pushed towards interventions that are totally unnecessary without understanding what they are signing up to. Their babies are being forced out of the womb before they are ready, leading to harm and trauma that have the potential for lifelong repercussions. Whilst I wouldn't disagree that a certain level of monitoring in pregnancy can be helpful and reassuring for those who choose it, we have to recognise that not all tests and checks are 'offered' in the best interests of the mother and/or baby, but more to eliminate the potential of the care provider being found negligent. I describe it as a 'tag, you're it' scenario. If, for example, a midwife measures you with a tape measure during a routine appointment and the size of your belly does not measure in line with the percentile curve you have been following, then they have to signpost you for a scan. In the past, medical staff would have requested to see you again in a couple of weeks, and re-measured, which worked just fine. These days, however, they pass you on so that the responsibility for your well-being and that of your baby is no longer in their hands. When extra monitoring is offered late in pregnancy, the appointments can expose you to the possibility of hearing negative comments and threats of birth complications or stillbirth, leaving you frightened and confused. Whilst any appointment offered is optional, it can take a confident person to decide not to attend. If you do decline, the best-case scenario is that your wishes are respected, but more likely, you can expect to be made to feel irresponsible. You may receive a telephone call from a doctor who will question your decision and perhaps coerce you into accepting more checks and monitoring. It's not unusual for someone to make appointments for you that you are not even aware of and certainly have not consented to. I don't say this to scare you, but to support you in being well informed.

Ultimately, if you do decide to attend any appointments offered, I recommend that you go feeling well prepared. It is important to write down any questions you may have for the doctor and be clear in what you want to say. After all, you do not have to justify the reasons you want to give birth in a particular way—it's your body and your choice.

Always understand that:

- You can ask as many questions as you want and take as much time as you need to come to a decision.
- You can accept or decline any or all procedures offered.

- Scans performed can be inaccurate when it comes to assessing the size of a baby. A 15–20% margin of error isn't uncommon.
- Different people performing growth checks can get different measurements.
- Glucose tolerance tests are designed to be effective only between 24–28 weeks and are optional.
- A predicted 'big baby' is not a reason to offer an induction of labour.

Sadly, fear kicks in once a pregnant woman and/or her birth partner have been spooked by medical professionals discussing 'potential issues' that imply you are unable to give birth without assistance. It can then become very hard to ignore or go against a doctor's advice. Seeds of doubt can be sown in your mind about the dangers of remaining pregnant, and you no longer trust that your body is keeping your baby safe. You find yourself questioning nature, wondering if your baby actually isn't the perfect size to fit through your pelvis, or whether your placenta might indeed 'fail' at the last hurdle. It seems that doctors no longer trust that babies will come when they are ready. This overmedicalisation of childbirth has led to the preferences of your care provider being paramount. They insist that they are the ones who should choose when and how to end your pregnancy, by pumping you full of artificial hormones to bring labour forward, replacing those hormones you naturally produce and thereby overriding your body's instincts and your baby's. Before you know it, you are flat on your back on a bed, strapped to a monitor, unable to move or guide your baby out through your pelvis as nature intended. The discomfort caused by these restrictions is more likely to affect your ability to cope, and your options for pain relief begin to feel essential. The hormones that were suppressed during labour because of the drugs are delayed and have to catch up once your baby has arrived. This delay can have a huge impact on the bonding process and milk supply, affecting both you and your baby. There are many other issues that can throw your plans off course, which I will discuss in other chapters, but for now, I want you to know that this book will challenge the need for most interventions and highlight the fact that we need to remember to trust our bodies. My message is that when the body is in charge, very little will go wrong. It's also important that you as the pregnant woman understand that you are capable of deciding for yourself how you want to give birth—and you should be supported in your quest to do so.

## Safe Birth

Whilst I recognise that everyone wants a safe birth experience, with a healthy baby born into their waiting arms, there is no reason at all why that can't happen for the vast majority of pregnant women without another person intervening. You are not designed to be meddled with, poked and prodded, attached to machines, and assessed during these incredibly intense and private moments of your life. You are not meant to be strapped to a bed and surrounded by strangers. Your body prefers a quiet, calm environment, which helps you to relax and soften. In order to stay safe, you must feel safe. Oxytocin, the hormone required to stimulate contractions and help your cervix dilate, will only be produced in abundance if conditions are optimal—similar to the ones we need when making love: warm, dark, private, and quiet. Constant distractions and sounds lead to the production of the hormone adrenaline, which prevents you from relaxing enough to get into the zone. If you understand your hormones (see Chapter 2), you will know that when adrenaline is present, it will reduce or stop the production of oxytocin, leading to slow or no progress and a long and exhausting experience. Safe birth in physiological terms therefore becomes about listening in to your body and following its lead. By feeling well supported and having the ability to relax and let go of any tension or anxious thoughts, you will find it easier to slip into the wisdom your body holds and trust your instincts. This is what makes physiological birth safe. It is a much clearer way for you to know when something might not be going well and, if necessary, you and/or your care providers can then act appropriately.

## Nothing Normal about Normal

The chasing of a particular birth outcome, often called a 'natural' or 'normal' birth, has been spoken of widely in the media in recent times. The implication in much of the coverage is that anyone who wants to achieve a natural birth could be potentially putting their baby at risk for the sake of an 'experience.' I can only imagine how confusing it must feel to be pregnant and hear stories in the news that suggest that you, as the pregnant woman, can cause harm to your baby by wanting to give birth in this particular way—that you should feel selfish or foolish to even expect to have a positive birth. This message is often compounded by your friends, family, colleagues, and anyone else who might share their awful birth stories with you to prove that birth is dangerous or unsafe. Well-meaning loved ones might question the alternative choices you make, because they themselves had a birth that didn't go well and might wonder aloud why you think yours will be any different. There is also a common perception that since we have come so far with modern medicine, why wouldn't you want to use all the available drugs to make your birth pain-free and easy. Why won't you just listen to medical advice? Here is what's happening: everyone, including friends, family, mainstream media, and to some extent your care providers, are getting confused between a physiological birth and a managed vaginal birth. The two are incomparable. So whilst a baby might be born through the vagina, it is not correct to say that a pregnant woman had a 'natural birth' if: she received drugs to stimulate contractions; she ended up lying on her back in restrictive and very 'unnatural' positions; and/or she had her baby pulled out by forceps or ventouse because she was told when and how to push rather than following the natural urges her body would have normally produced. There is nothing normal or natural about any of these situations, but sadly we have begun to see them as such.

Throughout this book, I want to ensure that you fully understand the distinction between physiological and managed birth, because it is important to recognise why, when birth is managed, it is more likely to lead to a cascade of intervention. The end result can be a difficult or traumatic birth, with you being made to feel that any issues were your fault if you 'didn't progress well enough' or you 'were too tired,' when in reality the management element of the birth was more likely to have been the cause of any problems. It's important to learn the differences between physiological and managed birth, so that if you are determined to avoid interventions, you will have the confidence to advocate for yourself when making decisions. It is crucial that if you intend to let your birth unfold in its own way, you are not made to feel that the birth you are planning is dangerous, especially if you decide to go against medical advice. I want to separate the two in your mind so you know why it is no longer accurate to describe anything other than physiological birth as 'normal,' and that if you choose this option, you might have to speak up to get the support you need.

### Three Ways to Give Birth

Let's look briefly at the three different ways your baby can be born. When you and your partner have a clear under-standing of all types of birth, you will be able to make well informed decisions that are personalised for you, both be-fore labour and also on the day itself.

### 1. Physiological Birth

The term physiological simply means that the body is left to function on its own without interference from modern medicine. When it relates to birth, the term conveys that the process should be untouched, unhurried, and undis-turbed. The ingredients for a physiological birth would include many or all of the following:

- Waiting for the baby to be born in its own time
- Not having any methods of induction performed, includ-ing a cervical sweep
- Allowing birth to unfold without time constraints
- Adopting instinctive positions and relaxing between contractions
- Eating and drinking regularly
- Avoiding internal assessments (such as vaginal exams), which can trigger the cervix to close down
- Respecting a natural pause if it occurs at any time, but in particular around full dilation

- Waiting for the instinctive urge to push that comes when the baby is ready
- Expulsion of the baby with no guidance
- Allowing the mother to decide when to gather the baby to her
- Transitioning of the baby's blood through the umbilical cord with no pressure to clamp or cut prematurely
- Allowing natural separation of the placenta from the uterine wall

These are the tasks your body is capable of during the birth of your child. Anything that undermines or interferes with this process may alter physiology, and therefore the direction your birth can take. I want you to understand that you can, of course, skip elements of the list above and still achieve a physiological birth, but the points on the list are not equal in their status if you accept an intervention. For example, changing to a recommended position rather than an instinctual one is not quite on the same level as agreeing to a cervical sweep. Both can be classed as interventions, but one is about getting you comfortable, and the other can stimulate contractions before the baby is aligned and ready to be born. Similarly, if you compare birth management methods, choosing gas and air or a TENS machine, which can be accessed in any environment including home, won't have the same detrimental influence on the progress of labour as an epidural, which has to be administered in a main labour ward, with your baby needing continuous monitoring and you needing a catheter inserted. An epidural has an immediate effect on the physiological process, shutting off pain receptors to the brain and leading to a reduction in oxytocin. The side effects can include a longer labour; your pelvic floor muscles losing their tone; you needing guidance to push; your baby requiring assistance to be born; and a possible delay in bonding with your baby. Of course it's up to you whether to choose to have a cervical sweep or an epidural, but I want you to appreciate that any scenario where the body is meddled with overrides physiology and can change outcomes, often resulting in a longer and/or more difficult experience for you. Lots of new parents are often unsure why their birth didn't go to plan, and this is typically why.

Oxytocin is the key to physiological birth, and knowing the role this hormone plays within your mind and body will help you experience a safe birth without intervention, simply by understanding how to keep it flowing (see Chapter 2). Even if labour is long, with the right hormone production the body will do all it can to encourage the baby into an optimal position and help the birth to be as quick and as easy as possible, assuming there are no unforeseen circumstances—or you change your mind about giving birth physiologically. If at any time you decide you would like an intervention, or you feel a clear indication that one is needed, then you have a wide range of options available to you with support from your midwife or doctor. This is no longer a physiological birth; it is now a managed birth.

## 2. Managed Vaginal Birth (Medical or Holistic)

In using the term managed birth, I mean no offence to anyone who might have, or go on to have, a birth that includes interventions, either medical or holistic. However, in order to differentiate between a birth that is physiological and all other births, it is important to share the elements that change physiology, therefore making the birth a managed one.

First, as mentioned previously, anything you do to the body to bring on labour has the potential to change the physiological process that occurs during the later stages of pregnancy. You can, of course, still try your own interventions (holistic) or accept interventions from your care provider (medical), but you will at least be aware that the body may no longer be able to rely on the same instincts, production of hormones, or guidance from both your body and the baby, leading to a potential change in the pattern and timing of the labour you have. Second, once in labour, anything that is suggested to you or done to you physically is an intervention. This includes a quick vaginal examination to check progress or someone instructing you to begin pushing. If your body is not working independently, and you are being poked, prodded, or timed, that is management of the birth process. It's also worth mentioning that when you disturb and break the natural rhythm of labour, you shut down the mother's ability to feel and listen to her instincts and those of her baby to move in beneficial ways (see Chapter 3).

A managed vaginal birth can include:

**Pre-Labour**

- Cervical sweeps and any form of induction
- Any holistic therapies that will attempt to bring on labour, including aromatherapy and homeopathy
- Consumption of foods or products that aim to bring on labour, including castor oil
- Inversions and rebozo to encourage the baby into alternate positions

**During Labour**

- Constant questioning and analysing that disrupts the flow of hormones
- Recommendation of positions that are not instinctive
- Vaginal examinations, which can affect vaginal microbes and dilation
- Continuous fetal monitoring, which is often inaccurate and requires you to be on the bed, as every time you move the monitor falls off
- Purposely breaking the waters around the baby, putting you at risk of infection
- Drugs or fluids given to relieve pain, which affect the body or mind
- Assisted birth techniques such as ventouse, forceps, or episiotomy (a cut to the perineum)

I hold no judgement to anyone who chooses or plans to accept any of these forms of management. I have opted for many of them myself. Once you begin accepting interventions, however, you may experience the need for more. This is known as the 'cascade of intervention.'

### 3. Abdominal Birth (Caesarean birth)

Abdominal or caesarean birth is often thought of as the 'worst case scenario,' that can happen to you when things go wrong and your plans have gone out of the window. This is not the case for everyone, and many will find the experience incredibly positive. A small percentage of people who are truly scared of vaginal birth, or would prefer to avoid one, will purposely plan an abdominal birth—and some will require one due to a medical concern such as the position of the baby or the location of the placenta.

An abdominal birth can be lifesaving, either for the labouring woman, the baby or both. It is, however, still major abdominal surgery, and the decision to opt for one should not be taken lightly. Consider:

- There is a risk of infection or complications.
- Recovery can be hard and impact your postnatal journey.
- It can have an impact on all future pregnancies.
- It can have a long-term impact on your health.
- It can have a long-term impact on the baby's health.

There is no doubt that some of you, despite planning for a physiological birth, may go on to choose to accept an abdominal birth at the end of your pregnancy journey. The reasons will become obvious to you at the time. Here are some recommendations for you in preparation.

**1.**   Where possible have a planned abdominal birth on the day labour begins. Waiting until labour starts on its own means the baby is ready, the lungs are mature, and the right hormones will be released. Your care provider will probably tell you it's not possible, because they want to have a date booked into their diary—but it is. If everyone only had an abdominal birth when the baby was ready, it would make such a big difference to the journey for everyone and for the lifelong health of the baby.

**2.**   In the weeks before birth, sleep with some muslin cloths. Share them with your partner, other children, even pets. These cloths should be exposed to your skin, mouth, and home bacteria. From the moment your baby is born, these cloths can be wrapped around them to ensure they keep warm and help seed their gut with your microbes. If the baby is removed from you for any reason, the cloths will be incredibly beneficial in building their immune system. Explain to your midwife or doctor that if you cannot have skin-to-skin contact with the baby, you want the cloths to be placed on top of any towels or blankets used. This is essential for a baby who is born abdominally, as they miss out on microbes in the vagina, and are exposed to antibiotics which also wipe out any good quality bacteria they have received so far. The effects can be symptoms like thrush, poor sleep, and skin conditions like eczema. In addition, I recommend you purchase a good quality probiotic for both you and the baby to help replenish any friendly bacteria you may have lost.

**3.** Write a solid birth plan that outlines what you are prepared to accept during your abdominal birth and what you are not. Just because you are having an operation, it doesn't mean you can't be involved in any decisions during that time. This is particularly important if, for example, you would like skin-to-skin contact with the baby, because babies are often given to the partner while the mother is being sutured. If you feel skin to skin in theatre is important, insist that you always keep the baby with you.

### Knowledge is Power

My goal in presenting the five key principles is to help you explore what your philosophies are around birth—to develop your Plan A and then ensure that you are not derailed from your plan as is often the case. The more you learn and understand what your body is capable of, the more in control you will feel on the day your labour arrives. Understanding hormones is crucial, and this book will help you to learn how to work with yours, ensuring that labour conditions are optimal at all times. I want you to hold the power throughout your birth, so you can achieve a positive experience no matter how your baby is born. I am going to help you tune into and trust your inner wisdom to find the power within yourself. Look at this book as an instruction manual on how to discover that power. First, you will need to identify any fears or doubts stored in your subconscious mind and uncover any uncertainty you might have in your body's ability to give birth easily. I also want you to investigate what the people who will be supporting you believe about both you and the birth process. Do they have any underlying fears they need to work on? It is essential to prepare your birth partner, family, and friends, because the right support is key. You can then have complete control of your birth experience, simply by letting go and trusting in the support around you. Understanding your rights and being clear on the philosophies of the maternity services you are engaging with is also vital, so that you know how and when to advocate for yourself. Your care providers should be respectful of your wishes and help support you to achieve them. Your birth experience shouldn't just be a positive one. It can be so much more, and I want to show you how to make it incredible. One that supports and honours the wisdom that you have within and deepens your trust in your own body and your baby. This trust will enable you to tune into the natural rhythm of your body, without the interruption of any negative thoughts that could reduce or inhibit your levels of oxytocin. These ingredients are the secret to achieving a physiological birth.

**THE FIVE PRINCIPLES**

**Understand your hormones.** If you don't get hormones, you won't get birth. Educate yourself about the role of hormones and the physiological processes of the human body.

**Trust your instincts.** Your intuition is your best superpower; prepare your subconscious mind for belief in your body's ability to give birth, and rid yourself of any doubt.

**Prepare your birth partner.** Your birth partner can make or break the birth experience. Educate your birth partner about their role in the process.

**Know your rights.** Hospital policy is not law. Set very clear boundaries about the care you are willing to receive. Practice saying No!

**Trust your body.** When the body is in charge, very little will go wrong. Let your baby decide when it's ready to be born.

## The Five Key Principles

I am honoured to be on this journey with you. I am a big believer in the power that you have and the incredible body that is yours! I am excited to share with you all the tips and tricks that have helped me and so many of my clients achieve their dream birth. In the following chapters, I have outlined the steps that you can take in order to educate and prepare both you and your partner for a physiological birth.

Assuming you and your baby have no health issues, and there is no clear, personalised medical need to intervene in your pregnancy, then you can confidently say 'No,' 'Nope,' 'No, thank you' or 'Not right now' to any medical procedures offered to you. The only thing most interventions do is sabotage your birth experience and cause long-lasting health issues for you and your baby, so be sceptical of advice given to you by a stranger in a white coat who probably hasn't even fully read your notes and has no idea what will happen to you if their recommendations are carried out.

### Amelia's Story

*From the outset of pregnancy with her first baby, Amelia was labelled 'high risk' due to her BMI, despite being tall. Anyone could see that she was perfectly in proportion, but she ticked a box and was therefore monitored closely. During several hospital visits, a glucose tolerance test (GTT) was offered, which she confidently declined. When I began working with Amelia and her husband, we sat down to discuss her wishes for the birth. She wanted to be given the opportunity to have little or no intervention and was keen to use the birthing pool. In order to be granted permission, Amelia was asked to prove that she could get in and out of the pool without support to show that she was not restricted by her size. It was humiliating for her; anyone with an ounce of common sense could tell that she was fit and perfectly agile. Amelia understood that she needed to be confident in her own ability to achieve her dream birth, because it became obvious to her that her care providers were not. We spoke in detail about how to trust the process of giving birth, and how* her hormones would support her if allowed to flow. In the end, learning about how her body would take over and push her baby out when the time came was a life saver. On the day, Amelia declined every vaginal examination that was offered to her by the midwives who were on shift. Her labour advanced beautifully until she hit a plateau for a few hours, where she continued to produce contractions, but instinctively felt that her progress had not advanced. The midwives caring for her expressed more doubt in her by recommending she transfer out of the pool and up to the main labour ward, not allowing her the time she needed to finish dilating and for her baby to navigate the pelvis. When Amelia declined, and chose to stay where she was, the midwife became very analytical and questioned her sensations: 'Do you feel anything different?' 'Did that feel a bit pushy?' Luckily, Amelia was confident in her body and knew that the time was not right yet, so she never once felt under pressure to perform. When the Fetal Ejection Reflex did kick in, her pushing stage was quick and her baby was born easily and within a short time. If Amelia had not done the work in learning to trust the birthing process, and if her birth partner had not been on board with her choices, the experience might have been very different. In the end, her unwavering confidence in her body, the knowledge that medical intervention was definitely not what she wanted, and the support she was given from her birth team, was everything she needed to succeed in achieving the birth she knew she was capable of.

The information you read throughout these chapters should build on what you are learning about birth in general, and give you the confidence to decide what exactly you want to achieve and how to put that into action. There is no magic pill or secret; it's as simple as believing in the power of your body. We were built to grow another human being inside us and to give birth without assistance. The more you understand about what your body is going through, the more in control you will feel, even if you have been labelled with so called 'risk factors' as Amelia was. She didn't have greater superpowers than the ones you have.

CHAPTER TWO

# Understand Your Hormones

*If you don't get hormones, you won't get birth.*

Not knowing enough about the important role specific hormones play throughout the birth process can lead to you having a long and exhausting experience. Deepening your knowledge of the way hormones are produced will ensure that you fully understand what can cause labour to progress or, conversely, to slow or stall. Typically, the latter is where interventions are recommended and birth plans go out the window. Let's begin by having a look at the role hormones play in general, and then I will share with you more specific information that will support you in achieving your dream birth.

## Hormones During Pregnancy and Birth

We are not entirely sure what triggers the cocktail of various hormones that are released when a baby is ready to be born. We do know, however, that each of the following hormones play a significant individual and collective role in pregnancy by not only signalling your body to begin labour, but ensuring it progresses throughout the birth process and then finally continues into the postnatal period with bonding and feeding.

Here are the main hormones and their role in brief.

**Relaxin** brings flexibility to a woman's body in the later stages of pregnancy, making room for the baby growing inside. This hormone softens and widens the cervix, and loosens ligaments, bones, and muscles in the pelvis in preparation to open easily as the baby comes through.

**Progesterone** keeps the cervix tightly closed and prevents labour throughout pregnancy. Closer to the day of birth, it begins to decrease, allowing the cervix to start the ripening process of softening and thinning.

**Prostaglandins** prepare the cervix for dilation. The process can happen over many days independently of dilation, or it can happen alongside. Prostaglandins are essential hormones that work with oxytocin to ensure that the cervix is soft, thin and ripened, and ready to begin opening during labour. Oxytocin aids the production of prostaglandins, so the two are interlinked.

**Oxytocin** stimulates contractions, which will become stronger and more frequent as your oxytocin levels build and progesterone and oestrogen levels fall. The contractions draw the cervix upward and out of the way so that the baby can pass through. Oxytocin is an incredibly fragile hormone and can easily be diminished or switched off by environmental factors such as lights, sounds, smells, or conversation. Once it is flowing well, it can work quickly and effectively at dilating the cervix.

**Endorphins** are the body's own naturally occurring pain relief, released in response to the body working hard. Beta-endorphins are a reward and can induce feelings of pleasure and well-being. They increase over the duration of labour when oxytocin levels are at their highest, giving you pleasure and making you look and feel very sleepy and 'out of it.' At this time, you should not be disturbed. Endorphins peak right after the baby is born and can leave you feeling euphoric.

**Adrenaline** is responsible for waking you up when your cervix is fully dilated. You will receive a huge boost of energy around the exact time you begin to push your baby out of your body. As you enter into 'fight or flight' mode, you can look wide-eyed and incredibly alert, despite feeling sleepy only a few moments earlier. Becoming more vocal and physically active is a clear sign that adrenaline is being produced. You may start to vocalise any fears—acknowledging that labour is too intense and that you cannot go on. This is called 'transition.' Sometimes there is a lull between the time of full dilation and the arrival of adrenaline, often called the 'rest and be thankful' stage, and you may think that labour has stopped or stalled. But this is a physiologically normal part of the birth process and should be respected—and the rest taken advantage of!—rather than treated as a delay or a problem that needs to be fixed.

*Please note: Whilst adrenaline is an essential part of the birthing process, the only time it should be produced is at the very end of dilation. If it is present too early, brought on by stress or fear, it has the power to slow or stop the production of oxytocin, which inevitably slows or stops labour. This results in long and more difficult births—the exact kind where interventions are typically recommended.*

**Prolactin** stimulates growth and development of the tissue inside the breasts in preparation for the production of milk and increases over the duration of your pregnancy. At the time of birth, alongside oxytocin, prolactin will flood the body to help with bonding. Prolactin signals the breasts to begin producing milk and then releases the milk to the breast each time the baby suckles.

**Postnatal Oxytocin** helps you bond with your baby in the moments following birth. In addition, you require oxytocin to help your uterus begin to shrink down to its pre-pregnancy size and safely release your placenta from the uterine wall. Therefore, it's important to let adrenaline levels left over from the pushing stage fall, to enable your oxytocin levels to flow in abundance. As the umbilical cord pumps blood from the placenta back into the baby, and you enjoy some skin-to-skin time, the rise in oxytocin will stimulate your uterus and you may begin to feel powerful contractions once again.

These will continue until the placenta is out of your body. Whilst not all new parents feel an instant bond with their baby, the presence of high levels of oxytocin and prolactin are fundamental to the bonding process.

**Oestrogen** and **Progesterone** levels drop even further after the placenta has separated from the uterine wall. This enables an easy flow of colostrum: a high-density milk ideal for newborns. As the baby feeds, high levels of oxytocin and prolactin are released from the mother's pituitary gland, stimulating more milk production and bonding.

## Without the Right Hormones, There Will Be No Labour!

Whilst all the hormones listed play a very important role, I want you to know about the following three in more detail, and to consider how they might affect you personally, because they have the biggest impact on the physiology of labour and birth.

- Prostaglandins
- Oxytocin
- Adrenaline

### Prostaglandins

Prostaglandins are essential for the early stages of labour. The cervix must go through what is described by medical textbooks as 'cervical ripening.' The softening and ripening process will help the cervix to shorten, thin out and move round to the front so that it can then begin to open and allow space for the baby to pass through and into the birth canal. There is a lot of physiological work going on behind the scenes that needs to be acknowledged. This ripening process can be happening silently in the background without you knowing, or it can begin at the same point as your contractions. Essentially, the cervix needs prostaglandins in abundance to carry out this important element of the dilation process, and it takes time and patience. If you are aware that labour has started, try to rest and relax to conserve your energy for later in the journey. The secret to achieving your dream birth is to make sure that at this stage you do not attempt to rush the process. This means that you should not be trying to bring on labour in any way as it can disturb the balance of hormones and lead to a delay or complication further down the line. I will say this many, many times throughout the book as it is one of the biggest mistakes that people make.

As labour begins, you may start to see your mucus plug and/or bloody show come away, and you might also feel some early sensations, or your waters might begin releasing. Regardless of what is happening, your job is to relax and rest when possible. This will help to shut down your neo-cortex (also known as your thinking brain) and increase the production of oxytocin.

During early labour I recommend one of the following two options.

**1.   Your birth partner should stay out of your way as much as possible.** You might choose not to tell your birth partner that you are in early labour, as it will make this stage much easier for you if you don't have to enter into any conversations about what you are feeling or experiencing this early in the process. If labour starts in the middle of the night, let your partner sleep so that your oxytocin levels can build. Once you need support, you can easily wake them to be with you. If labour starts during the day, and they work close by, send them to work. If they are at home, ask them to spend time in a different room, so they are not watching and waiting for you to progress, as this can subconsciously put you under pressure to perform, which introduces adrenaline and slows labour down. Staying away from each other can avoid you having to engage the part of your brain that will analyse and overthink, as it's inevitable you will end up chatting to them about your sensations and how you are feeling. Shutting down your analytical thoughts as much as possible is essential to ensuring that you are able to produce high levels of prostaglandins and oxytocin, thereby increasing your chances of a shorter labour.

**2.   Your birth partner can be present, but ONLY if they can help raise your oxytocin.** They must love you through the early hours unobtrusively and silently, nurturing you with hugs and kisses and softening you into the process. They need to ensure that your mind is clear of thoughts and keep all timers and analytical gadgets away. I would also recommend that you do not alert members of your family or engage on social media during this time. At this stage you have no idea how long you will be in labour, and if you have notifications on your phone pinging, people leaving responses for you that you want to read, and loved ones worrying about you and wanting updates, I guarantee that there will be a direct impact on your hormone production.

### Rest, Rest, and More Rest

The early part of labour, known as the 'latent phase,' is the period of time when contractions can vary in frequency and length. It is so important that you recognise this as a time for sleeping or resting and conserving energy as much as possible. If the conditions are right, and you are feeling safe, warm, and comfortable, then oxytocin levels will rise and you will begin to produce contractions and progress. You can eat something delicious and nutritious whilst drinking plenty of water to hydrate your body—this is important as your body is working hard and needs energy and fluids to function. Frequent trips to the toilet are recommended, as it is important to empty your bladder regularly to ensure the baby has as much room as possible to move down. Advice given by midwives at this stage often includes having a warm bath and taking a couple of paracetamols, but I recommend you avoid both if possible. Many of the over-the-counter pain relief remedies that you may have at home can prohibit the production of prostaglandins, which are essential at this stage, so any reduction is likely to lengthen your labour. If you would like to have a bath, I recommend lying on your side rather than your back. Lying on your back can increase the chances that your baby will turn to a posterior position, with their spine in alignment with yours. This is called a back-to-back labour and can cause you a lot of discomfort as your baby rotates in your pelvis trying to align. The start of labour is a very delicate time, and it is essential to avoid performing actions that you believe will bring on contractions. Any attempt to accelerate labour at this point, before your body or baby is ready, can lead to a long and exhausting experience. Rest, rest, and more rest is all that is needed, so getting comfortable by lying on your side or leaning over cushions or a ball is ideal, as you can then soften and relax all your muscles between contractions.

*Please note: Sitting or bouncing on a birth ball is not restful enough and can exhaust you. If you are trying to speed up labour in any way, you are not working with your body; you are engaging your thinking brain, and this will slow your labour down.*

## Oxytocin

Oxytocin is the queen of birthing hormones. It is required to produce contractions in the first and third stages of labour. Oxytocin has a few nicknames, including 'hormone of love,' 'cuddle chemical,' and 'the hug hormone,' because in order to secrete it, a person needs to feel loved and safe. In addition to its appearance during labour, you are likely to produce an abundance of oxytocin when you are surrounded by your friends or family, eating a delicious meal, playing with kids or pets, and during sexual arousal and orgasm. At all of these times I would expect you to be happy and enjoying the moment, rather than feeling stressed or anxious. It's the same for labour. You will naturally begin to feel sensations when you are calm and relaxed, possibly asleep, or when your mind is occupied with an enjoyable and engaging activity. Once it begins, the production of oxytocin is controlled by a positive feedback mechanism. It is initially released when a trigger occurs, in this case, your baby is ready to be born, switching on the hormone that produces contractions. As each surge makes the uterine muscles contract, your body pushes the baby towards your cervix, causing the cervix to stretch. This then sends a signal to your brain to produce more oxytocin. Initially, as your levels begin to rise, you may experience irregular contractions. Some might be short, others longer, and the gaps between can be random. In most cases, without high enough oxytocin levels, your contractions can be less effective. As time passes however, and with the right environmental conditions, your oxytocin levels should increase. As the feedback loop takes over, you will then see more consistency to the contractions as they begin to regularise and lengthen. This is a clear sign that you are producing high levels of oxytocin. As long as the body continues to receive the trigger, it will create more and more of this amazing hormone. For the loop to be preserved, you will need to experience many or all of the optimal conditions that oxytocin requires. The more you produce, the more your body will make.

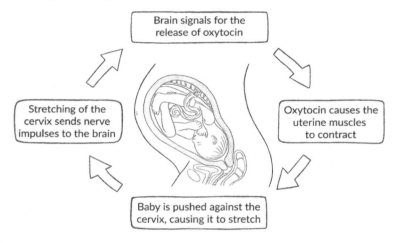

Brain signals for the release of oxytocin

Stretching of the cervix sends nerve impulses to the brain

Oxytocin causes the uterine muscles to contract

Baby is pushed against the cervix, causing it to stretch

## Raising Your Oxytocin Levels

Oxytocin is produced in copious quantities when you feel **safe, loved, warm,** and **comfortable**. It is no coincidence that labour often begins at night when you are in a **quiet, dark**, and **private** environment. The key to producing high levels of oxytocin once labour has begun is to **relax** and stay in the optimal conditions listed above. Surround yourself with familiar items that make you feel particularly safe, snug, and secure. Below are some items and ideas that you can use in any environment as well as take with you if you transfer to a midwife-led-unit or hospital.

- **Pillows that smell like home.** I recommend trying to fit two pillows into one pillowcase to make it more dense and therefore more supportive to lean on and relax into. Choose a pillowcase that is coloured or patterned so it doesn't get mixed in with the white hospital ones.
- **An eye mask.** If the room is too bright, you will produce less oxytocin and labour can take longer. You may close your eyes, but light can filter through your eyelids and still affect you, so close the curtains or blinds and consider wearing an eye mask.
- **Relaxing background music.** I recommend you prepare a playlist in advance of the birth and listen to it regularly. It should be so familiar to you that you can switch off your thoughts and become lost in the music. If you are using hypnobirthing tracks, then hopefully you will have listened to them numerous times in preparation. If you would feel more comfortable using headphones, then have them nearby. Noise cancelling ones are perfect for birth, especially if the environment around you is busy.
- **Soft blankets.** These are useful to cover you up and keep you feeling warm and cocooned. Blankets can offer a sense of privacy, but can get soiled later on, so don't use ones that are expensive or important to you as they may get disposed of after the baby is born.
- **Pleasant scents or fragrances.** Essential oils like lavender, lemon, frankincense or blends that are safe for

pregnancy can help you feel calm and relaxed in labour. You can use an aromatherapy system, or simply place some on cotton wool or tissue and keep nearby. I sometimes put 6 drops in a bowl of water and soak a flannel, wring it out and place on the back of the neck, forehead or lower back. This is the quickest way to get the essential oils to diffuse through the skin and into the body.

- **Focal points.** Sometimes it is helpful to have an image to look at that gives you a sense of peace and calmness. A focal point can be anything like a scan photo of the baby, a holiday snap, a few words of affirmation or an image of a loved one that is familiar and can help you to feel safe and relaxed.

*Please note: If you want to buy a string of battery lights to use during labour, make sure they are warm white and not bright white, as the blue light emitted from bright white lights can overstimulate the brain.*

## Adrenaline

Adrenaline is the hormone your body produces once you are fully dilated, to help wake you up from your sleepy relaxed oxytocic state, helping you to be fully alert and ready for the pushing stage. As I previously mentioned, despite adrenaline being needed in abundance at this point, it is important for you to remember that if it arrives too early, it can affect your labour dramatically due to its countereffect on oxytocin production. If you come out of your 'oxytocic bubble' just by feeling cold, or uncomfortable, by overthinking or overanalysing, being asked questions, or feeling unsure or unsafe at any time during the first stage, you will produce adrenaline. When labour is long and slow, it can be hard to put your finger on why it is happening. The impact of a long labour can really take its toll on you and leave you feeling exhausted. Your birth partner therefore needs to be the guardian of oxytocin (see Chapter 4). It is their job to shield you from as much outside stimulation as possible, and also take note of what your behaviour is like. You should not be timing your contractions and talking about them (how long or how often), chatting about your labour in a way that shows you are trying to control it or bring it on before it is ready, or look as though you are struggling to stay calm and relaxed. A huge red flag for your birth partner to look out for is if you are raising your shoulders and tensing, are unable to focus on your breath, or even thrashing around and/or making high pitched sounds. In my experience, a labouring woman who has high levels of adrenaline tends to appear as if she is trying very hard to relax, but in reality, has one eye half open all the time and is hyper-alert and unable to switch off. Look together ahead of time at the key concerns that you might experience on the day: fear, doubt, overanalysing of progress, lack of privacy, discomfort, too much sound or light, too many questions. For some, even being told to relax in itself can produce more adrenaline. So, it is important for you to be really honest with your birth partner in advance of labour and talk to them about how they can support you in any situation where you are feeling tense, anxious, or too aware. Your birth partner needs to know exactly what might cause an adrenaline spike within you and help you to avoid that where possible.

## Oxytocin's Enemy

Adrenaline is the enemy to oxytocin and can dramatically affect your birth. If you are overthinking and too present in your labour, adrenaline will be released, and your oxytocin levels will be knocked out by this powerful hormone entering your system. If your oxytocin levels do begin to lower, this will cause your endorphin levels to also drop off. As a result, you may start to find the experience of labour more painful and unmanageable. In this common situation, you can have enough oxytocin to be producing contractions but not enough to help your cervix dilate. You may be convinced that labour is advancing as your sensations feel intense, but I can guarantee you that in this scenario, progress is unlikely to be made. This is by far the worst situation to be in, because you will become tired and disheartened, and all hopes to give birth physiologically at this point can go out of the window, diminishing your oxytocin production even further. If the loop stops completely, and the body does not continue to produce oxytocin at all, interventions may be recommended. Understanding how to let go of thoughts and stay calm and relaxed in order to keep adrenaline at bay is therefore essential to ensuring you succeed in achieving your physiological birth.

## Jennifer's Story

*Jennifer called me at 8 am. to say that she had been labouring for about 5 hours. I asked her how she was feeling, and she said she was excited. She told me that her husband was staying home from work and that they had made plans for their friend to pop over. I knew in that moment that Jennifer would not have the baby that day, and it would be later that night before labour finally took hold. It wasn't until 9 pm, when it was dark outside and Jennifer was alone for the first time that her labour began to ramp up. She started to feel intense contractions by about 10.30 pm and she knew that things had shifted. At our debriefing session a week later, we spoke of how her labour had taken a while to get going, and she admitted that whilst she thought her friend would provide a welcome distraction, in reality, she could see that she felt observed by everyone around her. As the day progressed and her labour didn't, she began to overanalyse what was happening. As soon as she told her husband she was off to bed for an early night, her thoughts and expectations diminished, and her oxytocin levels rose, leading to stronger contractions.*

### Eliminate Excitement

It is particularly important in the early stages to try to eliminate any excitement if possible and to hunker down and rest. It is not uncommon to be so delighted the baby is coming that your adrenaline levels build, and contractions taper off and stop. I highly recommend you avoid any excitement at this point and keep away from physical activity like walking around or bouncing on a ball. You are far better off getting comfortable and adopting positions that help you to soften and relax your muscles, like lying on your left side, or leaning forward over the edge of your sofa. I always encourage my clients to 'plan for the long haul,' which helps you conserve all your energy for later. You will know if it is working, because as the hormones build, your contractions will become longer, stronger, and more frequent, and if they don't, then something is stopping them. Getting you comfortable is important to try and switch off from overthinking. Ideally, you want the room you are in to be as dark as possible, and you want to avoid conversation. I understand that you might feel like chatting, but you do run the risk of turning your birth 'into a party' if you are in entertainment mode, and this is the very last thing you want to do. As previously stated, I recommend that you are left alone as much as possible in early labour and stay out of the eyeline of others as much as you can. I find that when a labouring woman feels too observed, they will begin to feel under huge pressure to perform and adrenaline will slow down the labour.

## Parasympathetic and Sympathetic Nervous Systems

Let's dive a little deeper into the way hormones are produced. When you are in a high oxytocic state, your parasympathetic

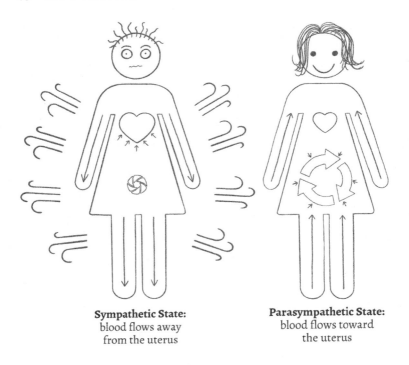

**Sympathetic State:**
blood flows away
from the uterus

**Parasympathetic State:**
blood flows toward
the uterus

nervous system is in flow. Otherwise known as 'rest and digest,' this state keeps your heart rate low, and blood flows away from your muscles towards your digestive and reproductive organs—in particular, the uterus. It can cause you to feel quite sleepy, easing you into that oxytocic bubble. In comparison, when you are producing high levels of adrenaline, your sympathetic nervous system is in charge—otherwise known as 'fight or flight.' Your body is prepared to run, so you are wide-eyed, and all your blood is pumping to your heart and limbs. These two divisions serve the same organs but create opposite effects in the body. They either excite your body's functions or subdue them. One ramps you up and prepares you for activity while the other talks you down, undoing what the other did. Our ability to enter 'fight or flight' when we are facing life or death is what has kept our species alive; if a sabre-toothed tiger came around the corner, we would definitely want all our energy to go to our brain, heart and muscles, or we would not have the ability to run away. Unfortunately, in modern times, our stress responses are triggered far too frequently as a reaction to our physical or mental equilibrium. This response can be caused by looming deadlines, financial issues, an argument with a loved one, or feelings of being overwhelmed. It is fair to say that many of us live in an almost constant state of stress, with the body barely ever getting a break. During the early stages of labour, even a small stressor can signal a problem to your body, and you will begin to produce adrenaline. As the uterus is not required or essential for the body to survive in a threatening situation, blood is therefore pumped away from it. This causes arteries going to the uterus to narrow and tense, restricting the flow of blood and oxygen. It's easy to see why labour might be slowed in this case. The ideal scenario is to be able to access your parasympathetic nervous system quickly and easily as soon as labour begins, so practicing relaxation techniques in the run up to birth is incredibly useful. It is hard not to feel some excitement when you know the baby is coming, but do your best to get into the zone as soon as possible. The deeper the zone, the faster your body can work—with no input from your brain. In such a deep effective state, the more you relax, the more oxytocin you will produce. This in turn brings on the contractions and enhances dilation. It's therefore important to recognise the parasympathetic nervous system as one of the key players in achieving your dream birth. Share this information with your birth partner so that they understand their role in the production of hormones (see Chapter 4), as this should lead to a shorter and more efficient birth overall.

### Hot or Cold Legs

When your parasympathetic nervous system is activated, and your oxytocin levels increase, your body will be working hard to produce contractions. Blood will be flowing away from your limbs to support your uterus, which can leave your feet feeling cold. This is why, if you look at recommendations of what items to pack in your birth bag, warm socks to stop your feet feeling cold near the end of labour will be near the top of the list.

One of the ways I try to identify if a woman is progressing during a physiological labour is to feel her feet and legs to see if the temperature has changed.

I tend to gauge it this way:

- If her legs are warm but her feet and ankles are cold, I assume her cervix is somewhere around three cm dilated.

- If her legs are cold up to perhaps the mid-calf area, she is probably around five cm.
- If her legs up to the knee are cold, she may be fully dilated.

**Please note:** *This method is not accurate if you have been using a birth pool.*

## Jess's Story

Jess was expecting her second baby and, with no signs of labour, was given a date for an induction at 42 weeks. Fortunately, she went into labour at 3 am the morning before. She arrived at the MLU at about 8 am and was shown into a room with a pool, which was in the process of being filled. The midwife told her that if she wasn't in established labour she would still be expected to attend her appointment with the doctor for the induction. This really upset her, and it's no surprise that during the time that midwife was in the room, Jess did not have a single contraction. I arrived shortly afterwards, and she was contracting beautifully, but sure enough, when the midwife came back into the room it all stopped again. The midwife became quite adamant that Jess could not possibly be in labour, stating she could only go by what she was seeing, despite our reassurances that she was contracting beautifully. I recommended that we swap to a different midwife, and while all that was being organised, I was able to get her into the pool. By the time the new midwife came into the room, about 20 minutes later, Jess was contracting consistently and showing signs that she was ready to push. The new midwife was shocked to discover this, as she had been informed that Jess was still in the early stages. She rushed around trying to get everything ready as the baby was born into the *water. In this situation, Jess's contractions were literally knocked out by the presence of someone who made her feel unsafe!*

---

## Traffic Light System

To end this chapter, I want to share with you the tool I use when teaching my clients the difference between oxytocin and adrenaline, to consolidate your knowledge on the role these key hormones play. I like to use the visual of a traffic light system to help demonstrate the damaging effects of having some levels of both hormones.

**Red = Stop.** When you are producing high levels of adrenaline, you cannot be in labour. That's because the powerful effects of adrenaline literally cancel out the effects of oxytocin. The body does not feel it is safe to give birth and so prevents labour from continuing. This can happen at any time in the process, if someone says or does anything to you that takes you out of a high oxytocic state, particularly if you feel frightened. A story I like to share is about a woman from my pregnancy yoga class who was expecting her third child. She was in labour and contracting beautifully. Her parents-in-law arrived to babysit her other children and her husband went and got her from the bedroom to help her out to the car. As she was leaving, she went to get her pillow and saw a massive spider on the wall. She froze as she was petrified of spiders, and in that moment her whole labour shut down. In the end, it stopped for four hours. She had to send her in-laws home and go back to bed and relax before the contractions returned and she was ready to leave for the hospital again.

**Amber = Contractions with no progress.** Once labour is in flow, your progress can be delayed by having some levels of oxytocin: enough to produce contractions, but also enough adrenaline to prevent dilation and delay progress. This means that you simply cannot dilate because your cervix is affected by the presence of any adrenaline. In all honesty, I would rather be producing high enough levels of adrenaline to knock out contractions altogether, and have a break, than have some levels of both and find myself stuck in a long labour where I was having consistent contractions, but not advancing. If you have ever heard of friends or family members who have described long, exhausting and debilitating labours, my guess is they were stuck in the Amber zone. They could possibly have been looking at their phones, contacting and updating loved ones on their labour, talking about what they were experiencing, and not getting in the zone and trusting in the process. This is a common story that I hear all the time. You can actively avoid a long labour, by NOT making the same mistakes.

**Green = Go.** Once labour begins, if the environment is safe and you are in the zone, then it will be obvious you are progressing. It is easy to observe that your contractions are becoming longer and closer together. Focus on your breathing at this time, in particular the exhalation, which may naturally deepen and lengthen. You will be aware that labour is getting tougher and may have short moments of doubt about your ability to cope, but you can move past these quickly by getting back into the swing of resting and breathing. When oxytocin levels are high, labour flows and your cervix can dilate.

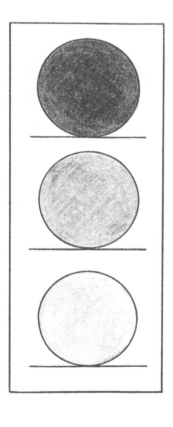

Red = Stop

Amber = Slow Labor

Green = Go

# *Summary*

- **Oxytocin and adrenaline are not compatible.** If your intent is to produce contractions and dilate your cervix, then you want to be producing high levels of oxytocin. Not medium or low levels, but high levels that continuously work to progress your labour.

- **Rest, rest, and more rest.** Despite the narrative that you will need to stay upright to get the benefit of gravity's assistance during labour in the early stages, it is more important for hormone production that you relax and rest, feeling safe and warm. Try not to do too much too soon, as you need oxytocin to build, and the best way to do that is to relax your body and your mind. The faster you can produce high levels of oxytocin, the quicker your labour will be.

- **Gather supplies.** Organise an oxytocin kit. What can you gather in preparation for birth that will help you in your production of oxytocin? You will need anything that supports you to feel safe, calm, warm, private, loved, and relaxed. Think pillows and blankets, relaxing music, eye mask, or essential oils.

# CHAPTER THREE
## Trust Your Instincts

*Your intuition is your greatest superpower.*

Understanding the role your instincts play in pregnancy is essential when planning a safe physiological birth. It's common to feel a little unsure about how to access this superpower if you have never tried before, but don't worry, your inner wisdom is definitely there ready and waiting. Just by exploring the idea of giving birth as naturally as possible you are already tuning into your instincts. Deepening your trust in your body's ability to grow and give birth to your baby without any external interference will help you succeed. It's common to struggle with expressing your thoughts, even if you already know within yourself what you want to say. You might find it hard to vocalise and share why you feel so strongly about the way you give birth—especially if your care providers are recommending interventions that you are keen to avoid. Instead of being listened to and understood, you can easily find yourself accepting these interventions and thereby overriding your own gut instincts. It's important to get really clear on the role this wisdom plays and how leaning in and trusting your body will help you feel overwhelmingly confident about your decisions. Do your research into the risks of all the procedures you want to avoid so that you feel well prepared. Then, if you do encounter a situation where a doctor or midwife is making recommendations, you can safely allow your instincts to flow, and have the research prepared to back you up. If you continually choose to decline medical advice, you will have the ability to overrule anyone who tries to diminish your plans. You should always believe in your innate wisdom above anything or anyone else, and if you are not able to speak for yourself, find an advocate who will speak for you. Learning to trust yourself is essential. Then you can discover more about the capabilities of your amazing body, by achieving a beautiful, physiological birth.

## Humans Are Placental Mammals

As mammals, our main purpose is to survive and pro-create. This involves growing, giving birth to, and feeding our young until they are capable of living independently. Humans fall into the category of placental mammals, which means your developing fetus is receiving nutrients and ox-ygen through the placenta, keeping it alive. The placenta is attached to the wall of your uterus and is joined to the baby via the umbilical cord. It enables your blood supply and theirs to remain separate and independent of each other. The placenta acts as the baby's lungs inside the womb, so they have no need to breathe until the moments after birth. As the baby's lungs transition in the immediate postnatal period, they start expanding, and the circulatory system changes to allow normal lung functioning to commence. At the same time, the umbilical cord begins to pulsate and the remaining 30% of the blood volume that resides in the placenta is vigorously pumped through, giving the baby all that belongs to them. As the baby slowly adapts from womb to world, your body will begin releasing hormones that cause your uterus to contract, allowing the placenta to separate from the uterine wall as your uterus begins to reduce in size.

As I highlighted in Chapter 1, this process all takes place with minimum fuss. So, whilst your midwife or doctor will want to check that your baby is breathing and will also be monitoring your blood loss, most of the other miracles taking place are overlooked and underappreciated. No one in the room is rushing around worrying about the extent to which you and your baby's bodies are adjusting in those vital moments. If we can trust the body for some parts of the journey, then why not ALL? Why is it assumed that some elements would fail and need assistance and others not? More credit should be given to the amazing job the human body does throughout the entire process, not just parts of it.

It's also important to mention that when other mammals give birth in the wild, they do not sit around feeling scared or frightened of the experience they are having. They seek privacy and are left undisturbed to give birth—with no interference from others—into less-than-sterile environments, where they can bond with their young without interruption.

There is a lot to be learned from the instinctive nature of other mammals. In their world,

- no inductions are offered;
- no one doubts their ability to give birth;
- no one is transferred anywhere;
- no assessments are made;
- no cervix is ever touched to check dilation;
- no one needs to guide them to push; and
- no one worries about the environment
  the baby is born into

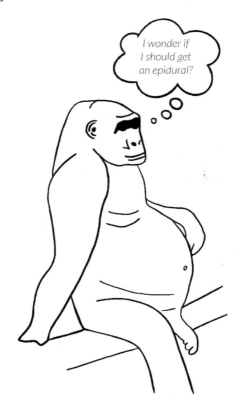

## Understanding Negative Bias

Did you know that humans have a built-in negative bias? This tendency to give more attention to what might go wrong has served us well as a species. It helped our ancestors to stay safe and evolve by alerting them to danger and keeping them vigilant of anything that might be a potential threat. Our negative bias protected us from harm, and those who were more attuned to danger were therefore more likely to survive. While we no longer need to be on constant high alert from the likes of a sabre-toothed tiger, research has shown that the negative bias we have in our DNA, passed down from those ancestors, still has a wide variety of effects on how we think, respond, and feel. The legacy of this bias means that when we hear negative news, we are more likely to perceive it as truthful. So, if you are watching TV or reading a post on social media that says anything remotely negative about pregnancy, birth, or parenthood, it is more likely to grab your attention and remain in your subconscious mind. This in turn fuels any doubts that may already exist in your subconscious about how dangerous birth might be. Similarly, if you have heard a horror story about a couple whose birth experience was traumatic, or where a baby died, then you are more likely to become heightened to any small issues within your own pregnancy. In addition, you will also be exposed to the negative bias that is carried by your relatives and friends based on the stories they themselves have heard. The influence that people who surround you in pregnancy and labour have on your birth plans can be dramatic, which can effectively shut down your instincts. You cannot be responsible for the feelings and fears that others may have, so it is important to state from the outset what you would like them to speak about (or not speak about) in front of you. Set boundaries and ask people not to talk to you about birth in a pessimistic way and stop anyone in their tracks who opposes your plans to give birth physiologically. This is not a time for politeness; it will help to minimise your exposure to fears around you. You can then tune into your own thoughts and feelings more clearly. You will be able to ensure that the only negative biases you hear are your true instincts. When you need them, they will keep you and your baby safe from the likes of a sabre-toothed tiger (or an unwanted and unnecessary intervention), and also alert you to a genuine problem—as long as you can shut out the noise.

## Care Provider Bias

What you cannot predict or be responsible for is any negative bias your care provider holds. You may have no idea what the person looking after you thinks or feels about physiological birth, but if they say something to you either in pregnancy or on the day itself that indicates they have doubts and fears about your ability to give birth in the way you are choosing, then you should consider changing to another health professional who is more supportive. Although this may feel awkward, it is vital that you have people around you that are respectful of your wishes. Don't buy into their misgivings about the human body. Your feelings of trust in your body must be so deep that you can override any words spoken in front of you that throw doubt on the physiological birthing process. During labour, again, if someone who is supporting you says anything at all that undermines your decisions about the birth you are experiencing, then asking them to leave your birth space is essential. This can be done firmly but politely, remembering that this is your birth, and you should only surround yourself with those that fully support you. Your partner may need to take them to one side and remind them to look at your birth plan (see Chapter 7). It can be a good idea for your partner to have their own copy of your preferences handy so they are easy to access and discuss. If necessary, they may need to speak with the ward manager of that shift and ask for a new person to provide you with care.

## The Power of Your Mind

Sigmund Freud described the mind as an iceberg.

**The conscious mind** at the top of the iceberg takes up approximately 10% and helps you to analyse and think. It contains all the thoughts, memories, feelings, and wishes you are aware of at any given moment. Your conscious mind can plan events, think of goals, or express feelings.

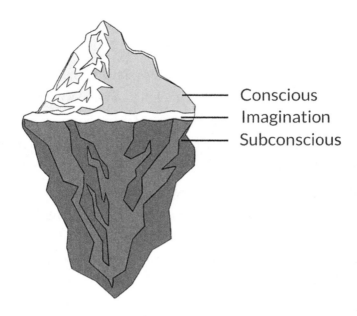

Conscious
Imagination
Subconscious

**The subconscious mind** is the remaining 90% of the iceberg hidden underneath the water. This is where you store repressed feelings, unconscious thoughts, fears, habits, desires, and reactions. It also stores deep-seated or hidden memories, including memories and emotions that you might find painful, embarrassing, shameful, or distressing. The subconscious mind exerts an influence on your daily behaviours and thoughts without you realising.

**The imagination** exists between the two—on the surface of the water. It links both parts of the mind, and communicates vital information when you need it, permitting memories or experiences to pop into your awareness during conversations to help with dialogue. When you are relaxed, your imagination allows you to daydream, think of brilliant new ideas, and access your intuition. However, your imagination also has the power to send information to the conscious mind that can lead to overthinking, worry, and negative emotions such as anxiety, fear, and frustration.

## Deep-Seated Thoughts

Any deep-seated negative thoughts lingering in your subconscious mind can easily begin to escalate in labour, causing the process to stall. For a physiological birth to succeed, and your body to produce an abundance of oxytocin and prostaglandins, it's helpful to eliminate any doubts, fears and negativity you may be feeling about the birth process in advance. You can then work on reframing the neural pathways in your brain by filling your mind with positive thoughts and images to overwrite those old negative ones. This will help you to remain in control of your birth on the day, as the deep knowledge and trust you have about your body's capabilities will ensure that if negative thoughts arise—which is likely to happen—you can remind yourself you are safe and strong, and the contractions are not more than you can handle. Then, you can confidently avoid many of the interventions that are available and often tempting to accept at this point. When your mind is filled with positivity, you will find it easier to relax and breathe and stay in tune with your instincts overall.

You will also want to identify what fears your birth partner may have, to ensure that you can reframe those to more positive ones. This will ensure that they are completely on board with the decisions you are making and will not be let down by any unwanted doubts or fears. The subconscious holds memories from before we were born, so it's impossible to imagine that you won't have any gremlins embedded in there somewhere. It might be from stories of your ancestors, from your own previous birth experience, from the TV, or stories from friends and family that you have heard over the years. Carmen Rocha, birth mindset coach and founder of The Birth Coach Company always says that mindset is everything when it comes to birth and beyond. She shares that success in achieving the birth you are planning consists of 80% mindset and 20% mechanics (meaning the position of you and your baby). Carmen says that when we are born, we are like little sponges, absorbing every thought and belief from our family, friends, and teachers. Her overall recommendation is that both you and your birth partner spend some time writing down your feelings about the birth process. Once you know what your fears are, you can move forward and work on reframing them.

## Reframing Your Thoughts

As you work toward a physiological birth, it helps to start reading information that supports your philosophies, looking at positive images, and talking to others who have given birth this way. Your subconscious mind will begin to absorb your preferences and recognise them as safe and effective. The calmer and more relaxed you feel, the easier it is to access your subconscious mind and begin to overwrite negative thoughts by replacing them with positive ones. These are the principles behind the popular practice of hypnobirthing. Once you begin to work on opening up the subconscious, you will notice an immediate difference and can start to see the positives everywhere you go. You can even write yourself personalised messages that you leave in familiar places, such as the dashboard of your car, the mirror in your bathroom, on the fridge door or as the screensaver on your phone. These messages are called positive affirmations and identify the beliefs you want to embed. If you have acknowledged any negative feelings about giving birth, these affirmations will support you to overcome any deep-seated beliefs you have. Rewrite them to reflect the positive messages you want your subconscious mind to know. Below are some examples.

| Negative | Positive |
|---|---|
| I am worried I won't be able to cope in labour. | I trust myself to breathe and relax during labour. |
| I am not feeling confident about giving birth. | I am strong and confident and I trust my body. |
| I don't want to lose control. | I will keep control by staying calm and relaxed. |
| I am scared I will find it hard to give birth. | I let go of fear, which helps my body give birth easily. |

What are yours? Perhaps you haven't any particular fears or you struggle to identify what you are feeling. You can just write down some positive statements such as:

*I am strong.*
*My body was made to give birth.*
*I trust my body completely.*
*I am safe.*

Or you might prefer words that encourage relaxation:

*Breathe*
*Relax*
*Surrender*
*Let go*
*I inhale peace and exhale tension.*
*I lengthen my outbreath instinctively.*

Whatever words feel right for you, write them down and ensure that they are placed in key areas where you will see them regularly. I also recommend you choose your favourite ones to use as focal points during your birth. Another idea is to practice saying the words or phrases out loud during your pregnancy. You could also record them or get your partner to record them onto your phone. Each time your subconscious mind sees or hears these words, you will know that they are working to produce new neural pathways in your brain that give you confidence in your body's ability to give birth smoothly and easily.

## Accessing Information Online

There is great power in reading and listening to information that supports the decisions you are making about physiological birth. I recommend you follow accounts with people who have the same philosophies as you. Even if you are not on social media, you probably have access to the internet, books, or podcasts, so you can access likeminded people who will help you to reinforce the message that birth works. It is important to try and listen to something positive each day. The more you surround yourself with constant stories and updates about achieving your dream birth—and hear about your body's amazing ability to give birth without medical intervention—the more confident you will feel if you encounter anyone who undermines that viewpoint.

Here are my recommendations for research-based information from medical professionals who support physiological birth.

**Dr Rachel Reed.** Rachel is the author of the blog *Midwife Thinking*; she is co-host of *The Midwives' Cauldron* podcast (with Katie James) and has written two books: *Reclaiming Childbirth as a Rite of Passage* and *Why Induction Matters*, both of which I highly recommend. Rachel also has an excellent online physiological birth course and is incredibly passionate and knowledgeable, sharing research-based information. You can follow her on Instagram **@midwifethinking**.

**Dr Sara Wickham.** Sara has written many books and each one is valuable when planning and preparing for a physiological birth. I particularly recommend her recent book *In Your Own Time*, which helps the reader understand the importance of allowing a baby to come when they are ready. All her books and resources can be found on her website at **sarawickham.com**.

**Dr Sarah Buckley.** Sarah talks about physiological birth and the importance of hormones and bonding. I highly recommend her book *Gentle Birth Gentle Mothering*, and I would also recommend her website **sarahbuckley.com** for supportive information.

## Biomechanics

Women's experiences during labour have been transformed over recent decades by discovering and understanding how their baby navigates through the bony structure of the human pelvis. When Janet Balaskas first wrote *Active Birth* in the 1980s, sharing her knowledge of labouring in upright, gravity-assisted positions, it revolutionised childbirth for those who read the book or attended her classes. Midwife Jean Sutton and antenatal teacher Pauline Scott wrote *Understanding and Teaching Optimal Fetal Positioning* in 1996, helping to change practice from the inside, by teaching midwives and other practitioners how the baby can rotate in the pelvis. This information supported women regarding movement in labour in order to influence the position of the baby.

Gail Tully's Spinning Babies® extends this concept, which Gail says is 'a paradigm of physiological release rather than mechanical,' helping women to understand that fetal rotation can be made easier if the mother knows how to make appropriate adjustments if or when the baby is not coming quickly and easily. The same can be said of Molly O'Brien's work with biomechanics, helping families and care providers look at the physiology of the pelvis and diagnose when a baby might not be in an optimal position—and know what to do if it's not. This information is arming women, midwives, birth keepers, doulas, and antenatal teachers across the world with tricks and manoeuvres that can be done in the event a problem is identified. So, as part of your birth preparation I recommend you become more familiar with your body and some of these concepts. It is important to be able to tune into any symptoms you feel, and then begin to recognise where you might need to relax and release more. Look up 'belly mapping' to understand what position your baby might be in and become familiar with their movements. Identify exercises that focus on relaxing areas of discomfort—such as the psoas muscle, which runs through your pelvis and can often be tight, causing low back or leg pain—and seek treatments that release your fascia (connective tissue), which can also be tight and lead to muscle pain. As an example, if either of these body areas remain tight when labour begins, it can cause a delay and sabotage your plans to give birth physiologically. If you discover ways to become more flexible and open, and understand the mechanisms of your pelvis and how to create as much space within for your baby, you can relax knowing you have given them optimal room to find the right position.

## Positions for Labour and Birth

Once you understand biomechanics, the way your body moves in labour should then be entirely instinctive for a physiological birth to be optimal. Nothing should be too prescriptive or planned out. You should have the ability to adopt positions that your body moves into intuitively, assisting the baby in navigating their way through your pelvis as easily as possible. Learning a variety of positions in advance of birth is useful, so that you get an idea about what feels comfortable, and what positions help you to rest and relax, using your own furniture at home in those early stages. This will help you recognise which positions work best for you, and which do not. There are a wide variety of resources you can purchase online showing ideas for the types of positions that can help create maximum room in your pelvis. I have included my recommendations in a downloadable document that you will find in the resources section at the back of this book. Share these positions with your birth partner so that they know how to support you to change position if you feel uncomfortable and want help. Get as familiar as you can with these positions, so that when the time comes you can let go of pre-set ideas about positions and just lean into what your body is guiding you to do on the day.

*Carly's Story*

Carly was 42 weeks pregnant with her first baby when labour started. Her contractions were uncomfortable from the outset, and she felt them all in her back. She told me, 'the only way I seemed to really be able to get comfortable was to lie upside down on the bed with my feet resting on top of the headboard to take the weight off and ease the pressure on the base of my spine.' What Carly was describing was an inversion. Because she thought lying on her back was bad for her, she chose to override her instincts and lie in a different position that was considered more 'optimal.' Throughout the night the contractions continued but as morning came and she lay down on her side to rest, they would ease off. This happened for three nights in a row, and looking back, Carly feels her body had been clearly trying to encourage her into the inversion position to enable her baby to turn. As she wasn't following her body's lead it meant her baby took longer to change position and she experienced several days of prodromal labour (stop/start). Eventually, Carly was so exhausted after 3 nights of no sleep, she finally agreed to an induction of labour. When relaying the story back to midwives since then she has been told that "in a long latent labour like that, especially with such protracted contractions, it's likely the baby was in the wrong position and needed more time to move round."

## Follow Your Body

When positions come from a place of instinct rather than direction, they are never wrong. So, whilst I invite you to learn more about the capabilities of your body, I want you to always remember that these recommendations are there for your use, only in case of emergencies.

Phrases like 'active birth,' for example, do not mean 'bomb around all day and exhaust yourself by staying active.' The meaning behind the active birth movement has always been to teach women to follow their bodies and move intuitively—to realise that lying on your back in labour restricts space in the pelvis and prevents your sacrum and coccyx from being able to move and open, that the extra space created can be as much as an additional 30% more room for the baby to pass through. You don't have to stand, and walk, and rock, and rotate in a certain direction if your body is telling you otherwise. This will exhaust you and most likely cause you to burn out before your cervix is fully dilated. It's not ideal to spend any time during labour lying on your back; however, sometimes women will choose to turn onto their back in labour because it feels right. This can be the same for any position that you might adopt and is especially true for the pushing phase. During this time, your body will help you to create space where it's needed. If you can move freely, you are likely to move your legs to facilitate more room in your pelvis in the best way for your baby. Acronyms like UFO (upright forward and open) and KICO (knees in calves out), are there to help you understand the movement your pelvis is capable of. The principle with KICO, for example, is when you draw the knees together as the baby is being born, you can open the pelvic outlet more. However, if your knees don't want to come together during the last stages of pushing, then leave them where they are, otherwise you could be causing more harm by prematurely closing off the pelvic inlet and trapping your baby. Don't force your body to adopt positions that you 'think' are optimal. Your body is far cleverer than that, and it will help to guide your baby out without you having to think at all.

The best way to find out what positions you like is to:

**1.** Practice some in pregnancy that will help you to relax and soften your body. Identify positions that are comfortable on the knees, the legs, your head and neck. Once each contraction has diminished you should try to let go of any tension and sink down into the position you have chosen. If you have a selection that work for you and help you to remain comfortable, then you might instinctively settle into one or two on the day without needing to think about it. It is important to remember that you should adopt positions in early labour that help you to conserve energy and rest. If you burn out too soon, because you were holding tension, then you might run out of steam before your baby is born.

**2.** Follow your body! So many times, I have witnessed my clients move instinctively in a way that no one could have predicted. Each time they were clearly moving to create more room for the baby, and they had no idea why. If you just let your body guide you, you will adopt positions that facilitate the right exit route for your baby.

3.   Gather your props. I take mats to go under the knees, a pillow to go under the buttocks, a peanut ball to open the pelvis, a pillow to rest your head on, a blanket to offer warmth and privacy, a flannel to make you nice and cool if you feel hot, and a bendy straw to enable you to drink plenty of fluids without moving your head. What do you need to gather to make your birth positions comfortable?

4.   Teach your birth partner what you like, so that if on the day you are struggling to remember, and you feel you need support, they will know how to help you. If they are able to use pillows, peanut balls, or birth balls to get you into a position that helps you relax, then you will be able to sustain the position for longer.

5.   If labour is long, and it becomes obvious that you would benefit from a change in position to encourage the baby to turn, then look at websites like **spinningbabies.com** and **optimalbirth.co.uk** that support biomechanics for birth. They can give you tips on how to turn a baby who might not be in an ideal position during a long labour. I recommend the 'Side Lying Release' and 'Forward Leaning Inversion,' both from spinningbabies.com. These are two examples of

ways to offer your baby the opportunity to adjust their position, by creating space within your pelvis, helping them to turn or tuck their head.

## Watching Birth Videos

It is helpful to research the type of birth you are planning by watching how birth unfolds when left undisturbed. Many of the images in your subconscious mind are probably based on the vision of women giving birth on their backs being directed by medical professionals. In order to reframe your mind to see birth positively, it can be helpful to watch beautiful physiological births. Let's imagine that your dream birth is in a water pool. Then watching lots of lovely oxytocin-filled water births to see how you would like to be treated can be helpful when preparing for your undisturbed birth. You will get ideas about your partner's role, what the environment might look like, and witness sounds and emotions that other labouring women experience. Equally, you might also see behaviour that you don't want for your birth, perhaps from care providers or birth partners who offer instructions or recommendations. Watching these births and learning what you do and do not want, will help you to write your birth plan and communicate your wishes to those providing support to you on the day (see Chapter 7).

*Lara's Story*

*Lara had a reasonably quick birth with her first baby. She progressed well and spent a long time leaning over a chair in an upright, gravity-assisted position. During the pushing stage, Lara got onto the bed and leaned over the end but wasn't comfortable. Just before her baby was born, she instinctively flipped over onto her back and pushed out her little girl. It troubled Lara for a long time that she had given birth lying on the bed on her back, because she knew it wasn't considered a 'good' or optimal position. I reminded her that when she spontaneously turned over, her baby was born within a few minutes, so for her it was a 'good' position because she was following her body. The same cannot be said for someone who is being directed by others, laying on their back strapped down by monitors, unable to move with their pelvis fully restricted. This is no longer instinctive and can cause more discomfort and lessen the space in the pelvis.*

## Stay Hydrated

It is incredibly important to stay hydrated throughout pregnancy. Your body needs extra water as it is busy making amniotic fluid, producing extra blood, building new tissue, as well as carrying nutrients to your baby and flushing out waste and toxins. You also need to drink plenty to try and avoid symptoms like urinary tract infections, constipation, headaches, heartburn and indigestion. Plus, including more fluids in your diet from food or drink can help prevent the pregnancy condition pre-eclampsia by keeping your blood pressure stable, and will positively affect your mental health by helping you feel better overall. Towards the end of pregnancy, it is important to remain hydrated in preparation for labour. This way you will know that as you enter labour, your body will be in an optimal condition. Keeping your fluid levels up throughout, is also important to improve the production of contractions, and because most labouring women burn off fluids rapidly, you will need to replenish by continually drinking as much as possible and remembering to empty your bladder regularly.

## Diet and Nutrition

A healthy diet is important throughout life, but during pre-conception and pregnancy it is essential. Eating the right foods to support the body is vital if you are planning a physiological birth. If you were not aware of the importance of good nutrition, it's never too late to change your diet and introduce more protein, healthy fats and good quality fruits and vegetables. My advice is to eat a wide variety of different foods that will give you as many nutrients, vitamins and minerals as possible. This will ensure the microbes in your gut are diverse, giving you optimal health and making you more resilient to external pathogens. Take care with soft foods like strawberries, nectarines, tomatoes, peppers, and cucumbers. They will need washing more thoroughly with bicarbonate of soda or apple cider vinegar before eating to remove any toxins from their skin, so when eating these foods, buy organic whenever possible. Foods like avocados, cauliflower, cabbage, pineapple, or melon that have a thick skin or outer coating don't absorb pesticides as easily, so are cleaner. Look online for updated versions of the Clean 15 and Dirty Dozen food lists.

Try to balance your meals to include protein, fat, and carbohydrates rather than having too many carbs over-whelming your plate. This helps to stabilise your blood sugar levels throughout the day. Two excellent resources for infor-mation on nutrition in pregnancy are 'The Brewers Diet,' which you can find at **drbrewerpregnancydiet.com** and **lilynicholsrdn.com**. Lily is a registered dietician/nutrition-ist who has devoted her career to researching real food nu-trition for pregnancy. She also supports pregnant women who want to prevent a diagnosis of gestational diabetes, and those who have already been diagnosed. As Lily states, 'most prenatal nutrition advice is outdated.' and her book *Real Food for Pregnancy* is essential reading for anyone planning to conceive—and *all* pregnant women.

## Health and Wellbeing

Looking after yourself can feel pretty instinctive during pregnancy. The first trimester teaches you to rest if you are exhausted, the second trimester shows you how to grow and adapt to your changing body, and the third trimester shows you how to bond and prepare for the arrival of your baby. The more you tune into your growing baby the more instinctive you can begin to feel as you learn to deeply trust your body. It is essential for a physiological birth to lean into that trust, knowing that your instincts will guide you, if and when necessary.

Your body goes through many different changes and stresses during this time, and one way to connect inward is to invest in some holistic treatments that support the body as your pregnancy develops. I recommend any or all of the following:

- **Pregnancy massage** with a specialist works on the lymphatic system, reduces cortisol, and relaxes tense muscles.

- **Bowen therapy** works on muscles and importantly your fascia, the thin casing of connective tissue that surrounds and holds in place every organ, blood vessel, bone, nerve fibre, and muscle, helping your body to stay in balance as everything shifts and moves as the baby grows.

- **Osteopathy** and **chiropractic** are slightly different, but they both work on posture and alignment as well as relieving symptoms caused by pregnancy such as pelvic girdle pain, sciatica, and sacroiliac pain.

- **Acupuncture** is an amazing treatment to alleviate symptoms like morning sickness, depression, and lower back and pelvic pain. It is also known for helping support you at the end of pregnancy to encourage your baby into an optimal position for birth.

- **Reflexology** helps to maintain balance in the body during the fast-changing emotional and physical changes you go through. By stimulating pressure points on the feet, it can improve circulation and alleviate symptoms like anxiety and stress, morning sickness, and low back pain. It can be used during labour to decrease the intensity of any symptoms felt, and the duration.

If you prefer, you can learn about ways to massage yourself at home using safe products or oils that will help keep your skin soft and supple as it stretches. There are lots of videos online that will show you massage techniques that you and your partner can use to stimulate your fascia (connective tissue) and keep it healthy, flexible and supple. I recommend including a daily tummy massage each day. Simply rubbing and touching your belly, perhaps talking to the baby as you do so, will help you connect with them emotionally. You may even feel them respond to your touch as they move and wriggle under your hands. You can encourage your partner to touch your belly, too, because not only can it be very relaxing for you, but it is a great way for them to bond with the baby. I also recommend you take time each day to walk out in the fresh air, as it is incredibly beneficial to build up your stamina in preparation for birth. The fitter and more flexible you are, the easier you will find your labour.

## Pregnancy Yoga

I highly recommend you attend a pregnancy yoga class if you have one nearby. The classes will offer you a dedicated time each week to focus on the pregnancy and tune into both yourself and your baby. This will help you to become familiar with your body and learn what you need as it adapts and adjusts. It will be easier to lean into some common sensations of pregnancy that you may not have heard of before if you know that others are experiencing them, too. As your baby grows and develops, your centre of gravity shifts, so it helps if you can learn ways to manage this, as well as how to tune into your instincts more. Moving, flowing, balancing, and stretching all creates room in your abdomen, hips, and pelvis, so the modified postures you adopt during a pregnancy yoga class are all incredibly beneficial. You will learn breathing and relaxation techniques that will help you to sleep better and give you some tools that you can use in pregnancy, labour, and parenthood. Any opportunity you have to practice relaxation is important to ensure you are familiar with the ability to soften your body in preparation for birth and let go of your thoughts. Your baby will love it, too, as they listen to your deep rhythmic breathing and benefit from your calmness. Lastly, you will meet other women who are at different stages of their pregnancy journey, and you can discover what kinds of decisions they are making and what type of births they are having. This can really help you to develop your own philosophies of birth so you know you are on the right track.

## Learning To Trust Your Instincts

I think it is hard for many of us to imagine tapping into our intuition. To believe it's really there, hidden within us and ready to go at a moment's notice. Perhaps you have never stopped for a minute and given yourself time to tune in. Even if you haven't realised or acknowledged it, I'm confident you will have heard, thought about or even used the expressions 'I had a gut feeling' or 'I listened to my gut.' Trusting your instincts during pregnancy, and in preparation for birth, is essential. That's why it's one of my 5 key principles. It's not just you who needs to believe deeply in your innate wisdom; it's also important to ensure that your loved ones believe it too, especially if for any reason they hold a differing viewpoint about your options for birth. Not everyone will understand why you might be choosing a physiological birth, especially if they are unable to eliminate the negative bias that may be embedded deep in their own subconscious mind. This can prove to be really tricky, when what you need is unconditional support. In the next chapter, I will focus entirely on the role of the birth partner, as they will need to be on board and support your decisions. Anyone you trust enough to share your plans with needs to believe in your ability to give birth as much, if not more than you do. I recommend that any influential people in your life are exposed to information that supports the reasons why you are choosing to birth this way. If you have already had a baby, you might be seeking a physiological birth because you had a negative experience and possibly even a traumatic one. It is common for anyone in this situation to plan a completely different birth, often at home and sometimes without medical assistance. If this is how you feel, then with or without you realising it, your instincts are telling you that there is a better way: a way to ensure that you don't have to go through the same level of intervention you had last time. If you have ever been bitten by a dog, your negative bias helps you to remember to beware of dogs; the same can be true of the maternity system! So, even though your decisions might trigger loved ones, perhaps even more than you realise, you will have to stay strong and firm in your reasons for choosing the direction you want your birth to go in, and their fears are not yours to carry. If, however, it doesn't 'feel right' for you to be honest with your family and friends about your decisions, then it might be best to keep them to yourself. If your instincts are warning you that it doesn't feel safe to open your heart and discuss your plans, then don't feel it's necessary to tell others. This is especially important if they hold the belief that the intervention you received during your previous birth saved your or your baby's life, despite the more likely scenario that the opposite is true. Ultimately, as long as you can remember that your instincts are powerful, and giving birth is not something to be afraid of, you will be fine.

Also, as part of learning to trust your instincts, remember:

- **Due dates are nonsense.** Don't put any weight into the Estimated Due Date (EDD) you are given, because they are rarely accurate, and it's probable that you are going to give birth after that date. Going beyond your EDD can cause anxiety and pressure, and all that adrenaline can switch off your ability to produce oxytocin, with the constant questions, time constraints, and suggested visits to the hospital for monitoring. From as early as possible, give your family and friends a date a couple of weeks beyond the due date, so that you can reduce the number of phone calls asking if you have had the baby yet. The more relaxed you feel, the more you can trust that your baby will come in their own time, when they are ready.

- **Never chase your labour.** When labour does get started, leave it to flow in its own way, and never try to hurry it along. You should be aware that speeding up your labour is about giving birth with your head and not your body. I want you to be guided towards doing what is right for you and your baby physiologically, so performing actions that will accelerate labour can disrupt that process. Unless there is a real deep-seated instinct that feels right to you, it is best to leave it alone. If, for example, you were keen to get up and rock on a birth ball at 3 am with mild contractions, I would want to know if that action comes from a place of comfort and relaxation. Are you just feeling that it is the right place for you to be in that moment, or are you sitting on the ball to get things moving because you are desperate to get on with labour, and you believe that being upright is the fastest way for the baby to be born? This is so important, because one is working with your innate instincts and the other is working with your head. Oxytocin is less likely to be present with the latter, and labour could become long and exhausting. It is so important to know that chasing a labour is not a wise move.

- **You can override your care providers.** Unless you are planning a freebirth, one of the biggest dilemmas that you and your partner will face during labour is when to call the midwife out to your homebirth or make the journey into hospital or MLU. Many make the mistake of accessing care too soon and end up being sent home. If you are truly following your body, going inward and not timing or analysing contractions, then in my experience I believe you will know instinctively when you want to make the call and seek support. If you are discouraged from leaving and being told to wait, but you feel strongly that you are progressing and want to settle into your birth space and get comfortable, then you will have to override your care providers and go anyway. This is especially important if your labour is advancing, but you don't fit the standard pattern of contractions that midwives or doctors believe indicates you are advanced enough.

You should always listen to your body and your instincts above all else. When you do access care, I would ideally avoid vaginal examinations (VEs) that may give false or inaccurate information at this point. As a VE cannot predict when your baby will be born, you could run the risk of being sent away unnecessarily and end up giving birth on the way home. (Read more about these points in Chapter 6).

*Please note: Once you arrive, if you are told it's too soon but you feel safer being close, consider accessing the chapel in the hospital and stay there for a while. It is usually quiet and empty and relaxing to just be in a (non-denominational) spiritual setting at this time, helping your oxytocin levels to rise.*

## The Birth Pause

In the moments after your baby is born, you may not feel the need to reach for them immediately. It's perfectly normal to take a minute or two to gather yourself. It can be surprising to others in the room, and some women are put under pressure to hold their baby before they are ready. So, take your time picking up your baby if that feels right for you. This is a physiologically normal part of the birthing process. Some women feel guilty or as if they have no maternal instincts, and yet this is one of the most instinctive moments that you can ever experience. Whatever happens in the seconds or minutes after you give birth, just try to go with the flow and feel into what is right for you. Trust that you know what you are doing. If you feel the need to wait and not pick up your baby immediately, then that is the right thing for both of you. This innate wisdom within you should be honoured and respected. Lean into what your body and mind tells you at any given time, and take a moment to acknowledge the power that your instincts hold.

## Summary

- **Negative bias.** Be clear on who you surround yourself with, and what their philosophies are about physiological birth. Do they align with yours? If not, you need clear boundaries in place about the way they speak or behave in front of you. If anyone providing you with care shows themselves to be unsupportive, you will need to swap to another person who is more respectful. In some cases, this may require changing to a different hospital or place of birth.

- **Positions for labour and birth.** Your body, when left alone to give birth, will instinctively adopt positions that encourage your baby through your pelvis in the easiest way possible. You can trust that you will know how to move, and find the right positions for you, so let go of any pre-conceived ideas about the positions you should be assuming and follow your body.

- **Health and well-being.** I really recommend that you focus on your health and well-being throughout pregnancy, or at the point where you realise how important it is to take good care of yourself both mentally and physically. Eat well and drink plenty of fluids every day. Massage your belly and connect with your baby as often as possible. Stretch and create space within you to accommodate your growing baby and learn breathing and relaxation techniques to support you—not only for pregnancy and birth, but for the early postnatal period too. You will benefit enormously from your partner understanding these techniques and they will in turn be able to use some of these methods to keep themselves calm.

CHAPTER FOUR

# Prepare Your Birth Partner

*Your birth partner can make
or break your birth experience.*

The people you surround yourself with in labour can affect your experience in a multitude of ways. You should choose your partner wisely to ensure that they fully understand your philosophies on giving birth, as well as what you want to achieve and why. You will need them to step up to the role and prepare well during pregnancy so that they provide you with the level of support you require and can advocate for you if necessary. They need to be fully aware of how physiological birth works and how their role often includes standing back and leaving you alone for much of the time. Birth keepers call this 'being, not doing.' If they don't appreciate how important it is to remain quiet and let the hormones flow, they can disrupt the process and hinder your progress. You will require unconditional support in order to achieve a 'hands off' experience, so your birth partner needs to be involved in all elements of your planning and preparation, including: understanding the role hormones play; writing a birth plan; packing your birth bag; and much more. Some partners find this a little overwhelming, and they might not be 100% confident in their role. For this reason, many couples hire a doula or birth keeper to join their team. A doula doesn't replace your partner (unless you want them to) but are there as a confident advocate who is experienced and knowledgeable and can support both you and your partner. They are a familiar face whom you trust to arrive at your birth knowing exactly what you want to achieve after getting to know you both beforehand. They stay with you throughout as an experienced guide, and will help to deepen your confidence in giving birth the way you are planning, as well as providing hands-on practical support if necessary. You can find a list of doula directories in the resources section at the back of the book to help you search for a doula who is local to you.

## Choosing your Birth Partner

Most of you will already have considered who might be at the top of your guest list when it comes to choosing your birth partner, and for most of you, it will be the other parent of your child. Ideally you want someone who will relax you and definitely not stress you out or bring their own fears or anxieties to your birth experience, as this can have a huge impact on hormone production. If your local hospital will 'allow' more than one birth partner, and you are not working with a doula but know you would appreciate extra support, consider asking a family member or friend. If you do have an additional person joining you, it is important to consider the relationship both you and your partner have with them. Invite them to your birth planning sessions so that they can sit with you and discuss their role within your team. Prepare them thoroughly for what you want to achieve and be clear on the difference between their role and your partner's. Take great care to make sure that there will be no negativity or conflict in the room with you, as this will dramatically affect your experience.

If there is a particular person who is keen to be with you during your labour, but you know they are not a great fit, you will have to be clear and decline their offer of support. Well-meaning family members can be very excited by your pregnancy and, without realising, sabotage your birth plans by messaging and asking questions all the time. The pressure it puts on both you and your birth partners to keep them updated is really stressful and brings adrenaline into the room. I recommend, where possible, that you don't even let your family and friends know that you are in labour.

## Claire's Story

*Claire learned the hard way when her mum told her she wanted to be at the birth of her first baby. She knew deep down that her mum would stress her out, so she kindly explained that she wouldn't be invited. Her mum was disappointed but asked if Claire would let her know the minute labour started, so she could feel involved from a distance. As promised, Claire messaged her mum when her waters broke at 4.30 am and kept in touch with her throughout the day. Her contractions were slow and didn't really get going until it was dark outside later that night. By the time Claire was ready to go to the hospital, it was 6 am the following morning. She was exhausted and had had little sleep for two nights. Claire knew her mum was worried, and it played on her mind. As labour progressed into day two, her partner was able to update her mum, but had to leave the room to get a signal which was annoying and distracting. All that day, her mum had been messaging asking for updates, and it became a real problem right up until the baby was born. Claire admitted that if she could go back in time, she would have not told anyone that she was in labour, as it inadvertently put her under pressure to perform. Speak to your birth partner in detail about avoiding using their mobile phone during labour and ensure that they do not contact any family members or friends.*

## Birth Planning Sessions

I recommend you arrange at least one or two birth planning sessions with your partner and anyone else that will be supporting you, to take place around 32 and 36 weeks. If you are attending an antenatal course together, schedule one to take place before the start of the course, and the other once it is complete. During these sessions, you should openly discuss with your birth partner your thoughts and preferences about giving birth. If you have any fears or concerns, this is the time to voice them and come up with solutions together. Talk candidly about what you expect from them in order to help you achieve your dream birth, then you can feel confident that they will make a good advocate for you. They need to trust you and your instincts, and fully believe that you would never make decisions that would put you or your baby in danger.

Here are some potential questions to guide your discussion.

- What are your wishes or preferences for this birth?
- What are your worries or concerns? Be honest!
- What do you think might irritate you?
- What birth management techniques do you want to try or avoid—breathing and relaxation, hypnobirthing, tens machine, acupressure, gas and air, epidural, opioids?
- What comfort measures or important tasks can your birth partner help you with during labour and birth— touch or massage techniques, hypnobirthing, cold or warm flannels, documentation (photos or videos), communication with people outside the birthing area?
- What are your preferences regarding the following: monitoring of the baby, vaginal examinations, induction of labour (including cervical sweeps), abdominal birth, optimal cord clamping, placenta encapsulation, feeding the baby, skin-to-skin contact, vitamin K?
- If it becomes necessary, how would you like your birth partner to advocate for you?
- What do you need to know about them and their needs during the birth?

At your second session together, I recommend you talk through your birth plan and share with them your hard and soft boundaries (see Chapter 7). I also suggest that at this time you pack your birth bag. This will help your partner to know what you have available for them to use to support you, and why. They will need to know exactly where to find these specific items on the day, to avoid distracting you and taking you out of your zone.

## The PROTECTS Tool

Share with your birth partner my PROTECTS tool. This is an acronym I developed and have been teaching successfully for many years.

**P Positions**  Make her comfortable, ideally with her pelvis free from restrictions, which can create up to 30% more room for the baby to move.

**R Refreshments**  Encourage her to eat small snacks and drink fluids regularly, to keep energy levels up.

**O Oxytocin**  Make her feel safe and loved, and offer quiet, dark, warmth, and comfort.

**T Timing**  Focus on timing contractions only when absolutely necessary—and be discreet.

**E Environment**  Take charge of her surroundings by turning out the lights, playing music, and moving furniture to make her comfortable.

**C Calm**  Support her in using breathing and relaxation skills, hypnobirthing techniques, and affirmations.

**T Touch**  Use massage, sacral pressure, anchors, and acupressure—if she wants them.

**S Silence**  Be led by her but try not to talk if possible.

Its intention is to help birth partners remember all the relevant parts of their role. Each letter provides them with a wide range of information that they can use to guide you through labour and birth.

## P: Positions

Positions in labour are so important to the process of physiological birth. I like to work on an "if it ain't broke, don't fix it' policy. Therefore, whilst it's the birth partner's job to make sure that you are comfortable and in a position that will help you relax, I hope that first and foremost you will adopt these positions instinctively. If, however, you tell your birth partner that you want to move and change position, they can make recommendations to help you. I suggest you practice a few together in advance of birth, so that they know what you like. They also need to know why gravity matters: upright positions support the physiological birth process by creating up to 30% more space in the pelvis. These positions facilitate the easiest possible route for the baby on its way through the birth canal and can also encourage the release of more oxytocin, which is essential for dilating the cervix. Download a free copy of my birth position recommendations checklist from the link at the back of this book.

## R: Refreshments

Over the years, I have met many couples who had a very difficult birth experience first time round. When I have un-picked what happened during their birth, I typically discover that they didn't eat or drink during the entire process. In most cases they simply forgot and had not made the connection to the fact that without food and water, the body simply can't function well, so the labour became long and tough. In this situation, contractions can slow down or stop completely, which can lead the midwife or doctor to want to step in and manage your birth by administering synthetic oxytocin and/or IV fluids to bring the contractions back. Ideally, we want to ensure that this does not happen to you, so deciding upon a list of foods that you know will be easy to consume is essential. Your birth partner may need to coax you to eat small snacks regularly, but it is important that you do.

**Early labour.** In the early stages of labour, I recommend that you continue to eat and drink as normal.

**Established labour.** As labour progresses, little and often works well for most people. A spoonful of yogurt, a small slice of banana, a honey stick. Some people like to pack coconut water, runners' gel, chocolate, frozen berries, or jelly. Nothing too complicated, but it helps to remember that you are not aiming to eat a massive snack if you don't want to. You should just eat something regularly to keep you going and give your body something to burn off. Your birth partner needs to eat too, but remind them to consume foods that are plain or bland—nothing too stinky that will make their breath smell, as your senses will be heightened during labour. (Or pack a toothbrush and toothpaste for them.)

**What to drink.** It is very important that you keep hydrated during labour, as you will be burning off a lot of fluids. I recommend you buy a pack of bendy straws or a bottle with a built-in straw, and drink consistently. Your birth partner can place the straw to your lips whenever you need a sip, so you don't need to hold the drink yourself. Whatever position you are in, and particularly if you are resting and relaxing on the edge of a cushion or the side of a birth pool, you won't even need to lift your head. This helps conserve your energy and keep you in a high oxytocic state. Suggestions include water, isotonic drinks, coconut water, sugary squash (not sugar free).

*Please note:* *If Entonox (gas and air) is used during labour it will really dry out your mouth, so it is wise to have a drink of water at the end of every contraction.*

**Burping and vomiting.** During labour, it is not uncommon for you to feel very 'gassy' and burp a lot. Some will feel nauseous, and others will actually vomit. Typically, this may only be once or twice, and whilst it can happen at any point, it is more likely to be towards the end of labour nearer transition. If this happens to you, then sucking on ice chips can be helpful. Sniffing lemon or lemon oil or using CBD (cannabidiol) is also thought to help with sickness.

**Going to the toilet.** A full bladder can affect the baby moving downwards, so once labour becomes established, be sure to go to the toilet at least every hour or two. Your birth partner may need to remind you. As labour progresses and the baby moves down, you may feel like you need a poo. This is when the bowel is being squashed near the entrance of the rectum. If you haven't already emptied your bowels before or during the labour, some may be released at this stage, but it is typically only a small amount. Don't be surprised; this is physiologically normal and useful for seeding your baby's gut microbes during the birth process. Your midwife or doula will clean it up as a matter of routine.

## O: Oxytocin

The birth partner is responsible for protecting oxytocin so that labour can continually progress. The production of oxytocin is essential in creating contractions and dilating the cervix, and levels increase when a labouring woman feels safe, warm, and loved. A dark environment gives natural privacy, which is why many will begin labour in the middle of the night. This powerful hormone is very easily knocked out if adrenaline creeps in, which can slow the process of labour down. It is essential to talk to your birth partner in advance and identify ways they can help you if they notice adrenaline is present. Classic examples are overthinking, overanalysing, or an inability to settle down (see Chapter 2). Gather tools that will help you stay calm and relaxed and show them to your birth partner, explaining what you will use them for. Pillows, eye mask, headphones, essential oils, cooling fan, flannels/washcloths, homeopathy, positive affirmations: if you discuss what to do in the event that you are unable to relax and switch off, you can create an action plan to help you get back on track. This will help you achieve a quicker and more straightforward birth experience.

## T: Timing

When it comes to timing contractions, my top tip is don't. Many women and their partners accidentally sabotage their plans by focusing too much on timings and relying on gadgets like contraction apps, which can often cause you to engage with care providers prematurely. Calling in support too soon can cause you to have a longer and often more difficult birth overall. This might be because you are just not in established labour yet, so your midwife leaves or you are sent home feeling very disheartened, thereby depleting your oxytocin production. Alternatively, you end up with unnecessary interventions because you are receiving care too early. In addition, there is a terrible tendency to analyse labour far too much when you are timing sensations, and you can end up discussing potential progress with your partner. Questions such as 'Was that one longer or shorter than the last one?' 'Do you think they are getting closer together?' or 'Are they getting stronger?' puts you both on high alert all the time. This can diminish your production of oxytocin further, sending you down the wrong track. Remember the traffic light analogy in Chapter 2: where some levels of both adrenaline and oxytocin keep you in the amber zone. This means you are still capable of producing contractions, but are unable to make progress. Protecting your oxytocin is essential so that you avoid the amber zone and remain in the green. In my experience the clearest signs of progress are when your contractions become consistent and regular. You can't talk or think during each one, and you need time to recover afterwards. When these signs are clear to your birth partner, and you are saying you are ready for external support, then they can sit quietly for about 10 minutes, and make a note of what is happening. Even just seeing them looking at their watch can be off-putting, so ask them to stay out of your eyeline and avoid discussing the results with you unless necessary.

They are looking at the following:

1. **Length.** Each contraction should be lasting at least 45 seconds to a minute long.
2. **Strength.** You have to completely focus on your breath.
3. **Distance between.** Look for regularity and a consistent pattern.

**Length.** Most contractions at the start of labour last 20–30 seconds and will lengthen as the labour progresses. Short contractions are over pretty quickly, and you will feel perfectly normal and 'back in the room' at the end of each one. As the labour begins to ramp up, your contractions will become longer and last more like 50–60 seconds. This is a clearer indication that labour is becoming established. As the sensations build, you will begin to focus more on your breathing, and will need some recovery time at the end of each one.

**Strength.** It is very hard for any birth partner to know what is happening for a labouring woman regarding the strength of her contractions. If from the outset you are calm and relaxed, it makes it easier to witness the progression of your labour as your breathing will change and become more forceful. If however, you are caught up in the fear-tension-pain cycle (see Chapter 6) they might struggle to see the difference in your behaviour and assume that you are unable to cope with the sensations. From the outset, I recommend you adopt a comfortable position and breathe, resting between surges to conserve energy when possible. It will then become more noticeable to you both when your labour is ramping up. You will know instinctively that the contractions feel stronger, and your behaviour will begin to change. You will no longer be 'back in the room' when each contraction ends and will need some recovery time. As your birth partner sits quietly over those 10 minutes of silent observation, they should witness this very clearly. If they randomly asked you a question during this time, you shouldn't be able to answer them until the recovery time has subsided.

**Distance between.** The blanket recommendation before considering heading to the hospital or calling a midwife out to you at home, is typically at least 3 contractions in every 10 minutes, lasting at least a minute, for a minimum of an hour. This is just a guide, of course, and if your contractions are not fitting this pattern, but you feel instinctively like you are ready for support, then you can override this recommendation. If your birth partner is timing your contractions, tell them in advance that what they are looking for is regularity and consistency between each one. Over time, your sensations will start to form a noticeable pattern that you could set your watch by. If you are having short ones, then long ones, then back to short with gaps that are randomly spaced, then you are not quite there yet. You wouldn't be ready to travel into hospital if they are 2 minutes apart and then 8 minutes apart and then 5 minutes apart. If the contractions are not forming a pattern and coming reasonably regularly then they are not considered to be 'established' just yet. A good gauge is when there is a regular distance between them: every 3 minutes, say. You want the pattern to be consistent, with approximately the same distance between each contraction. In addition, don't forget to remind your birth partner to look for signs that you are totally focused on the surges and need a recovery period after each one.

## E: Environment

Hopefully labour will begin at home, so you will be in complete control of your environment during the earlier stages. If you are remaining at home for your birth, then nothing needs to change. If you are using a birth pool, then you can ask your birth partner to begin filling the pool in preparation for when contractions begin to grow in length and regularity. If this is your second or subsequent baby, you may decide to begin filling the pool earlier in labour, in case things progress rapidly. If you are planning to give birth in an MLU or hospital, and you would like to use water, be sure to ask your birth partner to mention it on the phone when they call. I often ask the midwife to start filling the pool in preparation for my clients arrival, which many are happy to do. In the event that you are in a regular hospital room with a bed placed in the middle, then you will want your birth partner to take control of the environment as soon as possible after arriving. Ideally, they should try and re-create the space to be similar to what you were doing at home.

This may include:

- Adopting a comfortable gravity-assisted position.
- Having a drink next to you and snacks handy.
- Switching off the lights.
- Playing music that helps you to relax and/or feel happy.
- Moving furniture around to accommodate your birth preferences. You can raise or lower the bed to change it from a bed to a more convenient piece of furniture that facilitates your comfort, like a chair shape for example (download the checklist from the link at the back of the book).

## C: Calm

Both you and your birth partner should be calm and relaxed during labour. It is not your job to worry about others around you. If you are unable to relax because your birth partner or care provider is stressing you out, then you may need to ask them to leave, and only come back into the room when they feel calm and relaxed. For labour to progress easily, you require the maximum amount of oxytocin around you, and no adrenaline. If you think that your birth partner is going to struggle, then I would recommend you hire a doula to support you both through your birth experience. If you are practicing hypnobirthing, then take time each day to perfect the skill of self-hypnosis so that you yourself can use this tool at any time and stay calm and relaxed in all situations. My top tip is to ensure that when each contraction has finished, you should rest forward and relax all the muscles in your body. Then lower your head or close your eyes and stay quiet. This will help everyone around you to stay quiet too, and a lovely relaxing, calm atmosphere will be the best environment for your birth space.

## T: Touch

I find that during an antenatal discussion, when I talk about touch to my clients, most are delighted to hear that they might experience a lovely massage or be held and softly stroked in labour. If you feel the same, then discuss this with your birth partner and share with them the types of touch techniques that might work for you. Any practice you do together in the antenatal period will allow you both to become familiar with the relaxation elements of touch, and it will feel natural to you when this is implemented. If on the day you don't like it and you change your mind, you can ask your birth partner to stop, simply by saying 'stop' or by raising your hand. Some people however, will always be clear from the outset that they do not want to be touched. If this is something you think you might feel, then it's easy to share that with your birth partner. If for any reason on the day you change your mind, which can happen, you can let them know by sharing how you are feeling. It's common to ask for a quick hug or to be held for a moment.

## Massage Techniques

Massage techniques release endorphins. Here are some popular strokes your birth partner can use between contractions to help you relax.

**Light touch massage** involves being stroked softly with the use of fingertips. Your birth partner can lightly stroke your neck, across your shoulders and down your back using one hand or both to create a lovely tingling feeling.

**Nerve strokes** involves using a little more pressure and being stroked down each side of the back. Your partner can alternate hands, and always keep one hand on your back at all times. This is lovely to do between contractions.

**Shaking the apples** involves using one clenched fist on each bum cheek. Ask your partner to make circles with their fists to shake or jiggle your buttocks. This can loosen any tension and relax the muscles in and around your hips and pelvis. It can also give you a bit of an energy boost.

The following techniques are particularly useful to use during a contraction, providing an action that can help alleviate the sensations or open the pelvis:

**Figure of 8** involves drawing a side-lying figure of 8 using one or two hands around the lower part of your back, providing pleasant pressure over the sacrum. Tell your partner if you would like them to use more pressure.

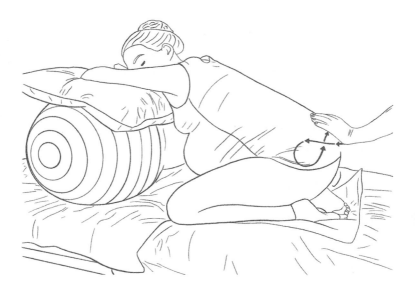

**Sacral pressure.** Using two hands, ask your partner to press all their weight into your lower back to relieve pressure in the sacrum. You might like them to put pressure on your sacrum at the start of each sensation, and then remove their hands at the peak if it feels too intense. Clear communication can help you get into a rhythm that feels good for you both.

**Double hip squeeze.** During a contraction, you might like your birth partner to lean in with their body weight and squeeze your hips together. This can help to splay open your pelvis at the outlet to create more room for the baby.

*Please note: If you are wearing a TENS machine for pain relief, it is much harder to use touch techniques for support. In this scenario, I recommend your birth partner focuses on upper back strokes, or strokes down the neck, shoulders, and arms to avoid touching the pads placed on your back.*

## S: Silence

It is important for you and your partner to remember that talking in the birth room can reduce the production of oxytocin. A common mistake is when you wake in the night with your first contraction and feel excited, so you share the news with your partner, or your partner stays home from work when labour begins and naturally wants to talk about it. The simplicity of entertaining each other inevitably turns your birth into what I describe as a party! These seemingly innocent actions can seriously delay your progress in the early stages without you realising. It is therefore always best to try and remain as quiet as possible, staying out of each other's way until labour is more established. If or when the time comes for you to engage with any care providers, they will understandably want to strike up a conversation with you as a way of bonding, by asking questions to you both. Whilst it may feel natural and harmless, again, the impact that constant conversation has on the birth process is far from innocuous and can add many hours to your birth. Even if it may not feel that conversation is reducing your oxytocin, because you are experiencing contractions, remember the amber zone in the traffic light. Progress may be slow, and this consistent chatter might be the cause, leading to an unnecessarily longer labour overall. Your birth partner should take note if you are becoming too engaged in conversation, because your goal is to go inwards. If they see that you are not, they will need to 'shut the room down' and make a point of staying quiet. They can encourage you to listen to relaxing music, or leave the room for a minute or two to break the conversation and then come back in and stay quiet from that point on. It is especially important for those who are providing care for you (midwives/care assistants/doctors) to respect that you would like them to be quiet at all times. Write this clearly in your birth plan (see Chapter 7), making it easier for your partner to remind all involved.

*Anja's Story*

*I went to Anja's home during the birth of her second baby. When I arrived at 3 am, Anja and her husband were both in their brightly lit kitchen, chatting whilst he emptied the dishwasher. Apparently, labour had slowed a little since she had called me to come over, and so they were just hanging out. I took a little bit of time to notice what was going on, and it was obvious that they were in entertainment mode and were asking me: Can I get you a drink? Do you want something to eat? What do you think we should do next? After about 15 minutes of catching-up time, I gradually began to reduce the level of my voice, and then suggested that it would be nice to go and get comfortable. I took her to the lounge, turned out the lights, put on some relaxation music, and stopped all conversation. Within 10 minutes, her contractions were back and within the hour she was in full blown labour. Her husband had inadvertently slowed her labour down by throwing a party in the middle of the kitchen at 3 am. If she had remained upstairs in their dark quiet bedroom after she called me, and he had gone downstairs alone, her contractions might not have slowed.*

## Lower the Tone

If you know from the start of labour that you would like everyone around you to be quiet, then make sure to lead by example. When you and your birth partner arrive at the hospital, or when the midwife arrives at your home birth, speak quietly from the outset. This will set the tone for the type of behaviour that you are looking for, and it is important to stick with that throughout. If a doctor or midwife enters the room and begins a conversation whilst a contraction is happening, always wait until the contraction has gone before you reply. Then always reply in a whisper. Don't be tempted to break this rule, as it can add many hours to your birth.

*Please note: It is not uncommon for a doctor or midwife to actually try and have a conversation with you in the middle of a contraction. In this instance, you should know that you can simply raise your hand and not attempt to answer them until you have recovered. Take your time.*

## The Marathon Analogy

Let's pretend you have signed up to run a marathon: something you are really keen to take part in. By signing up, you have made a big commitment, trained well, collected sponsorship money and bought all the gear. You have done a lot of research and have some set ideas about how you want the run to go. You have prepared both physically and mentally and have a running buddy to train with. As the big day approaches, you start to have doubts about your ability to finish the race. Even though you have been sure to surround yourself with people that encourage you and help you through, you have last-minute nerves. Your partner tells you that you are amazing, says goodbye, and watches you set off, agreeing to meet you at the finish line. As you run past them on the way, you are struggling. It's really obvious to them, but even though it is tempting for them to help you and shout out to you to stop and come home, they don't! Imagine how disappointed you would feel in them if they gave up on you and recommended you quit the race. You wouldn't want them to say things like 'There's no need to be brave! Just stop now and we can go to the pub for some lunch!'—of course you wouldn't! You are more likely to want them to run next to you and encourage you over the finish line with all the supporters along the way sharing words that boost your confidence and spur you on.

For some reason, when it comes to having a baby, many birth partners simply don't know how to help you to cross the finish line. Vocalising can scare them and make them feel unsure whether you want their help or not. The fact is that acknowledging you are struggling is a normal part of the birthing process for most women, so there is no need for your birth partner to say things to pacify the situation. They should simply keep you going—unless you 'safety word' them.

### Safety Word

A safety word is a special tool that I would not be without in any birth scenario. It is a word or phrase that is chosen before labour and can be used to indicate to your birth partner that you want to change your preferences, and switch from Plan A to Plan B or C. It gives your partner the added security of knowing that they can press on and support your wishes at all times, even if you look like you need or want them to step in and help. It is common for a labouring woman to vocalise during labour. You should feel comfortable doing this and know that your partner will understand this is normal. It is perfectly ok for you to find your current predicament tough and feel safe sharing your feelings, without them needing to 'fix' it for you. You may have moments where you doubt yourself, moments where you have a good cry, and you may have moments where you simply don't want to go on. What is important is that your birth team, whoever you have chosen, never gives up on you. You will always know that they have your back and are protecting and supporting your wishes during a 'wobble.' Sometimes an inexperienced birth partner can unintentionally say words that undermine your goal, simply because they want to help you. It's not uncommon for them to buy into advice from your care provider, who may lack knowledge about the physiological process of birth. So, the gift of a safety word means that as your birth partner, they can relax and feel confident in encouraging you to keep going with Plan A, even if you are voicing concerns. If you reach your limit, you will use the agreed word or expression and then they can help you make different decisions if necessary. Anything before that point must be one of deep trust. They have to trust in your body as much as you do. They have to believe in your ability to give birth as much as you do, and they have to be as strong as you are, so that even if you look them straight in the eye and say 'I can't do this anymore,' you know that they will confidently and calmly say 'You can, I'm right here, and you are doing great.' You can then vocalise as much as you want, and truly trust your birth partner. Then, at any point, if you use the safety word, they can stop and have a discussion with you about how you want to move forward.

If you do decide to step away from your Plan A, you will be making that decision for yourself.

Knowing a safety word is in place will:

- help you feel confident to vocalise as much as you want to.
- reassure you that your birth partner won't give up on you at any point because they feel secure in knowing you have the safety word in place.
- help all medical providers to understand that whatever happens, they should stick to your list of preferences unless you use your safety word (or a genuine medical need arises).

*Please Note: If you are using gas and air, and you say your safety word, it is important to have one or two contractions without using the gas. Your birth partner can then feel confident that you have clearly expressed your wishes, and that you will remember the conversation.*

## Being, not Doing

I want to end this chapter by sharing with you that the best possible birth companion is someone who can truly understand the concept of being present with you in labour—and not feel the need to do anything at all. If all is going well, they can sit quietly and observe. They should not try to 'fix' the birth for you, even if you vocalise and share that you are finding it tough. Always remember that when it comes to physiological birth, 'less is more.'

The PROTECTS tool is simple and easy to use, and a short-ened version is available as a free download with this book. Print it out and keep it handy for your birth partner to refer to on the day. Their main role is to ensure that you are calm and comfortable, getting regular snacks and drinks, and us-ing the toilet every hour or two. They should then feel confi-dent to sit beside you and do very little. If at any point during labour things change, and you require more from your birth partner, they will know how and when to step up and pro-vide you with additional emotional and/or physical support. At that point they can implement whatever you need in that moment, as you will have discussed your preferences and practiced some techniques in advance together at your birth planning sessions. Otherwise, a good birth partner will ben-efit by staying quiet, keeping calm, and resting when you are resting.

## Summary

- **Birth planning sessions.** Organise a couple of sessions where you are completely focussed on talking about your birth plans. I recommend one around 32 weeks and another after your antenatal course has ended at around 36 weeks. Turn off your phones and sit down with no distractions. Talk about what you want to achieve, how you want them to support you and how you would like your partner to advocate for you if it becomes necessary.

- **The PROTECTS tool.** This useful acronym will help your birth partner to know the important elements of their role. This will help them fully understand the relevance of each of the 8 points and apply them to the birth process. Go through them together during your birth planning sessions.

- **Safety word.** Choose a safety word, to give you both the ability to relax into labour knowing that your birth partner has your back. No matter how much you vocalise, their role is to keep you going with Plan A. If you use your safety word, then at that point, you can discuss Plan B or C and decide what you want to do next.

You will find more information to help prepare your birth partner for their very important role in my dedicated book *Labour of Love: The Ultimate Guide to Being a Birth Partner.*

CHAPTER FIVE

# Know Your Rights

*Hospital policy is NOT law.*

*Y*ou will only have each birth once, so it is important to
make 'this' birth the best that it can be, by taking ownership of your experience. Recognising the extent to which
the way you birth can affect both you and your baby will
give you an insight into why the decisions you make
around your options are so pivotal. Understanding the
difference between hospital policies and maternity care
guidelines is helpful, but the bottom line is that neither
can enforce you to accept any treatment or procedure that
might be recommended. Always remember that hospital
policy is NOT LAW—and you are NOT IN JAIL when you
enter a hospital to receive care. You can accept or decline
any procedure offered to you as an adult with capacity (a
person who is deemed capable of making their own decisions). It is your right to give informed consent or refuse
the recommendation of any examination, treatment or
intervention given by a midwife or doctor. Informed
consent is the fundamental ethical and legal doctrine
that protects the patient's rights of personal autonomy
and bodily self-determination. So, whilst a hospital can

make policies which can affect your birth options, for example withdrawing homebirth service, they cannot stop you from having a homebirth.

## The Reality

Sadly, whilst so many care providers working in maternity services know your human rights and are fully aware that they should gain true informed consent from you when making a recommendation, most don't. They are supposed to share the risks and benefits to any procedures offered and give alternatives that you can choose from, give you time to decide, and then support you in that decision. Unfortunately, it is common to find yourself attending an appointment with your midwife or doctor where they give you information you do not understand. You can feel really vulnerable, especially if you are presented with information about what is going to happen to you in a way that indicates you don't have a choice when you do. You might, for example, be told without discussion that you will be booked in for a scan appointment, or you might be informed you have to give birth at a particular time in your pregnancy. I've heard some classic stories: 'I had to have an induction because they thought my baby was big' or 'I wasn't allowed to have a homebirth because I had Group B strep' or 'My partner wasn't allowed to join me until I was in established labour.' Whilst common, not one of these examples are accurate statements and no information you are given about your birth options should ever come across as being set in stone. You always have a choice.

## Gaining Informed Consent

If you find yourself being told by your midwife or doctor at the hospital that you are 'not allowed' or 'not eligible' for any of the preferences you might have for your birth, and no discussion takes place about your options, then consider asking your own questions. You can use the popular acronym T-BRAIN to ask for more information that will help fill in your knowledge about the benefits, risks, or alternatives to any advice given. This will help you fully understand what you are being told, so you can decide if any recommendations made are right for you. You need individualised information, to be able to understand what you are consenting to. Also, any conversations you have about your options should be relevant to your current situation. This means that you shouldn't be expected to process information about inducing labour at 39 weeks when you are at your 20-week scan appointment. It is impossible to make well informed decisions when you have not had adequate time to learn and understand what alternatives there might be. Even if or when you have agreed to a plan with your doctor, you can change your mind at any point if it no longer feels right for you.

| T-BRAIN |
| --- |
| **T Time** Is there time to discuss my options, or is this an emergency? |
| **B Benefits** What are the benefits to the recommendations given? |
| **R Risks** Are there any risks involved to me or my baby? |
| **A Alternatives** Are there any alternatives to be considered before making a decision? |
| **I Instincts** What are my instincts telling me? |
| **N Nothing** If I choose to wait, can I change my mind at any time? |

## 'NO' Is a Complete Sentence

You might be surprised to learn that you can decline care, or that you have choices, although I hope by now you are aware that you can say 'no' to any or all recommendations made to you regarding procedures offered. I want you to always re-member that nothing can be done to you without your con-sent, and no one can touch you without asking permission. Saying no to a serious medical procedure can, of course, be up for discussion. There may be a good reason for your care provider to be making a particular recommendation to you, as long as they give you a balanced viewpoint. Anyone en-gaging with doctors wants to ensure they are given person-alised information that relates to their particular situation, so they can learn and understand the risks and benefits as well as alternatives. This will help if you find yourself in any situation where you might need to make a decision. Then, if you decide to say no, your decision should be respected.

Because so few women realise they can decline any element of their care, they are often made to believe that checks and procedures like the initial assessments performed in labour—which include invasive examinations—are not optional. A classic example is when you arrive at the hospital in labour, or when a midwife arrives at your homebirth, and they ask to assess you, they might assume they are gaining your consent by saying something like: *'I would like to do some initial checks and monitoring to see where you are—is that ok?'*

These checks typically include you getting on a bed and lying down so they can:

- check your blood pressure and pulse
- listen to your baby's heart rate
- feel your belly to check the position of your baby
- perform a vaginal examination to assess your cervix

The problem is that if you aren't made aware this assessment is optional, it is therefore not acceptable to expect you to comply and then call it consent. It is a criminal assault to perform a procedure on you of this nature without you fully understanding what you are agreeing to, especially when one of these checks is something as intimate as a vaginal examination. So, please remember that if someone expects to touch your genitals, which is an incredibly private and sensitive area, you have the right to say 'no,' 'no thanks,' or 'not right now' every time you are asked and you should not have to explain yourself and enter into a discussion as to *why* your decision is no. As birth rights activist Emma Ashworth always says 'you have as much right to put your fingers in your care provider's vagina as they do in yours: absolutely none at all!'

If, once you have declined, you are then exposed to coercive comments like 'it's safer to do an examination upon arrival' or 'our guidelines state we must do an examination', or the common one 'how will we know you are in labour if we don't check you' or worse still, 'we can't let you in the pool unless we know how dilated you are,' then you will need to ask your birth partner to step in and advocate. Anyone who is pushed into agreeing to an examination at this point is not giving full informed consent. If you choose to decline, your care provider should accept your decision and document in your notes that you have declined, without further conversation, except perhaps to remind you that if you change your mind at any point in the future, they would be happy to discuss your options further.

## Guidelines

**Guidelines** (noun): *A general rule, principle or piece of advice. Synonyms: recommendation, instruction, direction, suggestion.*

Each hospital works with a set of guidelines that have been decided upon by a multi-disciplinary team. In the UK, these are selected from recommendations provided by organisations like the National Institute for Health and Care Excellence (NICE), the Royal College of Midwives (RCM), the Royal College of Obstetricians and Gynaecologists (RCOG) and the Royal College of Paediatrics and Child Health (RCPCH). In addition, guidelines are influenced by the personal experiences of the physicians, and the needs of the local demographic. Any appointments or procedures recommended to you by your midwife or doctor will be based on these guidelines, so understanding how they will influence the care you are offered is important. You can then accept or decline all, or part, of any recommendations made, which will be documented in your notes. If at any point you are unsure of what you are consenting to, speak with your care provider so you can fully understand them in advance of making your decision. If, like many of my clients, your antenatal care provision is at your local hospital, but you have chosen to give birth in a different town where the services are provided by another, their guidelines are unlikely to be the same.

## What Do You Have the Rights To?

1. **You have the right to life.** You yourself have the right to life. Whilst this might not be true in all countries, in the UK your baby has no rights until after they are born. You have the legal right to make choices in childbirth, which includes the right to decline all medical care, even if this may cause harm to your baby.

2. **You have the right to humane treatment with no suffering.** This means that you have the right to be offered appropriate pain relief if you want it, as long as there are no clinical contraindications which could cause you harm by receiving the medication.

3. **You have the right to respectful care.** This includes the right to choose your place of birth, and who attends the birth with you. You have the right to bodily autonomy, which means that no medical procedure can be carried out without your consent. If your care provider fails to give you sufficient, objective, and unbiased information in order for you to make an informed choice, they are violating your human rights.

4. **You have the right to not be discriminated against.** You must receive equal treatment and not be treated differently because of race, religion, disability, immigration status or national origin. There are, in fact, 9 protected characteristics: age, disability, gender reassignment, marriage and civil partnership, pregnancy and maternity, race, religion or belief, sex, or sexual orientation. The Equality Act specifies that it is against the law for any NHS organisation or care giver to discriminate based on these characteristics. This does not mean, however, that everyone should be given exactly the same care. The law exists to ensure that someone who is compromised is provided with extra care and support, to enable them to be equal to anyone else who is having a baby.

5. **You have the right to freedom of thought, conscience, and religion.** This includes having the freedom to change your belief, religion, and thinking whenever you choose. Your beliefs should be respected and supported. This means you should never be forced to think in a particular way. Your right can only be interfered with if there is a need to protect the rights of others.

## Just in Case Medicine

Doctors who took the traditional version of the Hippocratic Oath used to swear to 'first, do no harm' when they completed their medical training. Understanding the body and its ability to work well in most cases meant that a doctor needed to offer treatment only when it was necessary. The words 'first, do no harm' have now been replaced with the words 'to do good' and 'not to harm'. Whilst I believe that anyone who provides care within maternity services wants every family they look after to have a positive birth experience, the truth is that many families are not. Far too many women and babies are receiving unnecessary medical interventions that are in fact causing both physical and mental harm. Their experiences are far from positive and, unbelievably, women themselves are blamed for any problems that arise during their birth, when it is more likely the fault of interventions they received. Doctors are even deciding to end pregnancies early to prevent the possibility of an unpredictable complication. They no longer trust women's bodies to keep babies safe and so intervene, for example, by giving synthetic hormones like Syntocinon/Pitocin. When care providers jump in and give synthetic hormones, they effectively suppress your own natural hormone production, leading to a long list of side effects. Without your own hormones being released to support you, there is a greater chance that you will choose pain relief medication. These additional drugs are well known to cause further intervention. For example, 50% of women pregnant with their first baby who choose an epidural will require assistance with forceps or ventouse. When the body is altered by these chemicals, it not only reduces your chances of having a straightforward birth, but can also have consequences in the immediate postnatal period by impacting your ability to bond with your newborn, and by increasing your longterm potential to develop postnatal depression. Iatrogenesis is the name given to the harm caused by these interventions, which come with physical and mental side effects that can actually place women and their babies in as much, if not more, danger than the reasons for the initial intervention. Incredibly, these alternative risks are often never shared or discussed, and your care provider may fail to give you the comparison between the effects of using drugs and not. So, whilst there are usually risks to either choice in a given scenario, these risks are yours to weigh and decide upon, not your care providers'.

The overwhelming fear that something 'might' happen to the baby during childbirth can cause more harm in the long term because of these interventions. Many children are being seriously affected by their difficult, long, and often traumatic birth experiences where they are pumped full of synthetic hormones and chemicals, the result of which typically involves them being pulled out of your body by their heads using rough hands or instruments. In addition, the more women's birth experiences are being meddled with, the fewer doctors and midwives are able to witness physiological birth. This has resulted in a huge gap in the learning process, and a deep lack of understanding and knowledge of the physiological needs of a labouring woman. With levels of interventions going through the roof, we are now seeing an abdominal birth rate of 40% or higher in many areas. It cannot be denied that something is very wrong within the current system and these 'just in case' philosophies of care are leading to deep harm! In this chapter, knowing your rights is also about understanding your responsibility in the decisions you make, and remembering that nothing we do in life is risk-free.

## The Montgomery Ruling

In 2014, a court in Lanarkshire, Scotland, heard Mrs Nadine Montgomery share the story of the birth of her child Sam, who sadly suffered hypoxic injuries and cerebral palsy due to shoulder dystocia (the baby's shoulder was stuck on the pubic bone during birth, leading to a delay). Mrs Montgomery was very small in stature, had Type 1 Diabetes and a predicted big baby, so was recommended to have an induction of labour by her consultant at 38 weeks. Mrs Montgomery had expressed concerns to her consultant that she might have difficulties giving birth to Sam due to his size, but the consultant was confident in his decision and the risk of shoulder dystocia was not discussed with her, or indeed any alternatives, including an abdominal birth. Her consultant said in court that he felt if he had shared the risk with her, she would have opted for the C-section, and he didn't believe this was in her best interest. He stated that the risk of shoulder dystocia was so low that it was not considered to be relevant, but commented that if she had asked, he could have shared the information. The argument in this case was that Mrs Montgomery had not been allowed to make a well-informed decision regarding her options for birth. The risks of induction were not discussed and no alternatives were given. She had never been made aware that the effects of lying on her back on a bed during an induction of labour could dramatically increase the risk that her baby might struggle to be born easily. This is a perfect example of iatrogenesis, where harm was caused by the interventions given.

At the ruling in 2015, Justice Brenda Hale stated: 'Gone are the days when it was thought that, on becoming pregnant, a woman lost not only their capacity, but also their right to act as a genuinely autonomous human being.'

The court further expressed: 'The law on consent has progressed from doctor-focused to patient-focused. The practice of medicine has moved significantly away from the idea of the paternalistic doctor who tells their patient what to do, even if this was thought to be in the patient's best interests. A patient is autonomous and should be supported to make decisions about their own health, and to take ownership of the fact that sometimes success is uncertain, and complications can occur despite the best treatment'.

## Fear-Based Practice

Since the Montgomery ruling, little has changed regarding the sharing of evidence-based information to ensure pregnant women have the ability to make well informed decisions. However, what has changed is that doctors and midwives have become more stringent in their behaviour. You are likely to hear words like 'shoulder dystocia' spoken, often unnecessarily during your routine antenatal appointments, without any additional or individualised information, and no mention of what the actual statistical risks are. So, don't be surprised if this happens to you. You can't sue them if they've documented it's been said! This fear-based practice is unhelpful and can leave you feeling scared and worried that your body will not be able to give birth to your baby easily, making you more likely to accept help. Care providers are still failing to recognise that by keeping information to themselves, they are effectively coercing you, so any decisions made at that point would not be informed consent, anyway. It's really no surprise that 50% of all hospital litigation claims are against the obstetric department.

## Understanding Risk

I'm not a huge fan of the word risk, but ultimately it is a word you are likely to hear at some point during your pregnancy journey. You may have been told from the outset which risk category you fall into as a way of determining the care pathway you are on. This then predicts how many tests, scans, or extra appointments you are 'offered.' At any time in your pregnancy, your care pathway might change, and a recommendation may be made for a medicalised birth when you had planned for a physiological one. In this case, only you get to decide if the change in your risk status means that you are no longer eligible for the birth you are planning. You—not your care provider—are the one who needs to weigh the risk to you and your baby. There are risks to everything we do in life: eating, sleeping, walking, driving, flying. When it comes to pregnancy and birth, no one will ever be able to give you absolute certainty that everything will be ok. Life and death are interwoven, and we cannot escape the fact that not all pregnancies will result in a live birth. So, whilst no one can give you a guarantee that your baby will be safe if you choose physiological birth over managed, the reverse is also true! A doctor or midwife can never say that the interventions they offer you will be safer than leaving well alone. There really is no such thing as 'risk free'; it's simply a case of understanding the risks of all options and deciding which one to choose. I want you to know and understand how to evaluate risk so that you can accurately decide what seems best for you in the circumstances you are in. Taking responsibility for weighing each risk might feel incredibly overwhelming, and it is ok to accept or decline the advice given to you from your care provider. If you are giving consent for any recommendations made to you during an appointment, then you are supposed to be presented with information that is clear and easy to understand. Whatever decisions you make about your pregnancy and birth options should then be documented.

### Material Risk

Discussion with any doctor is called a consultation and meant to be a two-way conversation. When you attend an appointment, you should remember that if risks are being discussed, there are many types. Material risk is a risk that is deemed to be of significance by an individual person rather than by a body of doctors. In order to discover what may concern a patient (or, in this case, a pregnant woman), it is imperative that the doctor endeavours to find out what matters to her. There can be no 'one size fits all' approach to any medical care. Documentation of this discussion and the options offered is important and is required by the General Medical Council (GMC). The GMC guidance states that the principle of involving patients in their treatment and sharing information with them about risks has been in place for some time; however, the Montgomery ruling didn't recommend only pointing out the risks! Instead, it advocated pregnant women being supported to make well informed decisions by not only helping them to understand any alternatives, but also by respecting their decisions. The ruling pointed out that it is the doctor's role to give the women they care for all the information required to enable them to make a balanced judgement between different options, and to document they understood the risks to all those options. A consultant obstetrician from a recent conference I attended reminded his audience of that by saying 'The Montgomery ruling has changed how we practice medicine. There is great pressure on midwives, sonographers and doctors to identify a suspected big baby, or gestational diabetes. You must give parents information about expectant management risks and benefits, induction risks and benefits, and c-section risks and benefits. You must share that information verbally and must document that discussion. You should then have access to a specific pathway as to how that should be done so that you don't feel pressured into giving the wrong information.'

This ruling was meant to change the way care is provided and make it more woman-centred. You should be able to expect a more active and informed role in treatment decisions, with a corresponding shift in emphasis on various values, including autonomy and medical ethics. If your care provider is not giving you all the risks, benefits and alternatives to information they share, they are letting themselves— and, more importantly, you—down. In this scenario, you yourself will have to ask for them.

## Relative Risk vs Absolute Risk

In most cases, when risk is spoken of in relation to pregnancy, you will likely hear information given to you as a relative risk. Your care provider might say words like 'I recommend this procedure because you are at increased risk of . . .' or 'In your case, the risk doubles.' Often this way of speaking is enough to scare you into consenting to the procedure offered, and you go ahead with recommendations made. This way of communicating risk offers no help with making a well-informed decision, so what you need to hear is more personalised information that is factual and useful. When it comes to achieving a physiological birth, you want to be able to look at your own individual circumstances and make decisions based on the absolute risks to you and your baby as individuals. If you have discovered a reason for medical intervention, and you are deciding whether to switch from Plan A to Plan B or C and accept those interventions that are being recommended to you, understanding how they affect you is important.

Megan Rossiter from **www.birth-ed.co.uk** explains the difference between relative risk and absolute risk really well by using the example of car colour.

**Relative Risk:** 'If you drive a black car, you're twice as likely to have a car accident than if you drive a white car.' This is a way of describing 'relative risk' and it's essentially useless information.

**Absolute Risk:** '2 in 1000 people who drive a black car will be involved in an accident. In comparison, 1 in 1000 people who drive a white car will be involved in an accident.' This is a way of describing 'absolute risk' and has the potential to give us a far better picture of what MAY happen. Additional information about the type and condition of the car, the age of the driver, how the accidents occurred, the weather conditions, and time of day would be even more beneficial in helping the purchaser to understand the true risk, so that they can decide which one to buy.

It is easy to be misled when statistics are given to you in a deceptive way. Technically, .2% is indeed 'double the risk' of .1%, but .2% is still incredibly low. Information shared with you that encourages important decision making should be given more accurately and include information that is personalised where possible. In addition, the risks of their recommendations should also be shared with you—in particular the risks of serious interventions being offered, like induction or abdominal birth.

Let's look at information your doctor might share with you if your baby is predicted 'big' (4.0 kg or larger) regarding the risk of shoulder dystocia.

**Relative risk.** Doctor: 'As your baby is measuring larger than average, you have an increased risk of shoulder dystocia, and so we are going to induce you at 39 weeks.'

**Absolute risk.** Doctor: 'There is a slight increase in the risk of shoulder dystocia occurring in big babies. Whilst rare, 52% of babies who experience shoulder dystocia are 4.0 kg or larger at birth. As your baby is predicted to weigh more than 4.0kg, we would like to offer you an induction.'

Although neither of these examples are particularly helpful and offer no personalised risk about your own individual situation, at least when given the absolute risk, you can see that the difference between a 'big' baby and all other babies experiencing a shoulder dystocia at birth is very small. If additional information were to be discussed, you would discover that the chance of your baby becoming stuck as it is being born is less than 1% and more likely to occur in babies born via induction. If your doctor had also highlighted that more than 99% of babies are born with no concerns at all, and your chances of success are increased further by avoiding induction—therefore allowing yourself to move freely, creating up to 30% more space in your pelvis—I'm sure you would be less likely to be concerned about any 'risk' of shoulder dystocia they felt they had an obligation to mention (since the Montgomery ruling). Their job is to carry out a discussion, giving you all your options and document your wishes once you have made a well-informed decision. They can support you in making that decision, but they should not be scaring you into interventions or making recommendations without giving you alternatives, as was the case for Nadine Montgomery. Let's compare the outcome of a client who accepts what she is told to one who questions everything.

**Client A** is 36 weeks pregnant and has just had a midwife appointment. After checking her fundal height measurement (the size of her tummy), her midwife is worried. She is 38 cm: two centimetres more than was expected, giving concern that her baby might be growing bigger than average. She is told she must go to the hospital for a scan to check the size, as a big baby is at an increased risk of shoulder dystocia. Client A was led to understand that there is an increased risk (relative) but was not made aware that the risk was very small (absolute). After the scan, a consultant told her that she had to have an induction of labour at 39 weeks due to the potential size of her baby, and a date was booked. Client A felt really worried about the fact that her baby was big and might get stuck during the birth, which played on her mind. In the end, the induction was long and took many days, and she struggled to relax throughout labour. With slow progress and her baby beginning to show signs of distress, Client

A had an emergency abdominal birth. Her baby weighed 7 pounds, 12 ounces, and was therefore not considered big at all. At no point had anyone ever shared with Client A the risks of induction or the risks of major abdominal surgery, despite the chance of complications for both of these interventions far outweighing the possibility of a shoulder dystocia occurring. In addition, the psychological effects it had on her were dramatic.

**Client B** is also 36 weeks pregnant and measuring 'big!' Her midwife tells her she must go for a scan to check the size of the baby. Client B asks some questions about her recommendation for the scan, knowing the fundal height measurement is just a guide. She reminds the midwife that she doesn't have to go and would prefer to decline the scan until she has done a bit more research. Client B discovered that scans cannot accurately predict the weight of a baby and can be out by as much as 15 to 20%. She didn't want an induction as it would affect her decision to give birth in the local midwife-led unit and increase her risk of an abdominal birth. During her research she also found on the Royal College of Obstetrics and Gynaecology website (rcog.org.uk) that shoulder dystocia occurs in only 0.5% to 0.78% of births overall, and that one of the risk factors was an induction of labour. Client B was reassured that her baby was the right size for her, and she declined any further tests or scans. She went on to have a wonderful relaxing birth in the pool on the MLU.

## Question Everything

By asking questions and doing her own research, Client B had a very different experience to Client A. By declining appointments and interventions offered, she avoided her birth becoming medicalised. She decided that the risk of shoulder dystocia to her baby was minimal. She also didn't expose her baby to harmful medication that caused distress and resulted in major abdominal surgery. Induction of labour is offered for a variety of reasons and often recommended at around 39 weeks with no conversation to the risks of complications from the induction. As well as the possibility of it taking many days to get you into labour, this procedure can increase your risk of additional interventions, including requiring an abdominal birth, which could not only have an impact on all future pregnancies, but increase the chances of your baby being transferred to intensive care.

Reasons given for an induction of labour might include:
- High BMI
- You are over 40 years of age (younger in some countries)
- Baby is measuring small
- Baby is measuring big
- IVF pregnancy
- Low Papp A
- Pregnancy has gone beyond 41 weeks
- Controlled gestational diabetes

- Your ethnicity
- Your placenta could fail
- Your last baby was big
- Previous shoulder dystocia

If you fall into any of the categories above and are being sent for extra tests, checks, or scans without discussion, if you are being told you will or should be having an induction of labour without the risks of induction being explained to you, if you are being told 'your risk doubles' or 'you are at increased risk' or if you have been warned that your baby could get stuck (shoulder dystocia) or die (stillbirth) if you don't agree to a recommendation—you will need to question the person giving you this information.

Here are some ideas for questions you can use:

- Could you explain that again, please, but also include the benefits and risks?
- Can we discuss what alternatives there are so I can make a well-informed decision?
- Is this your personal opinion or an evidence-based recommendation?
- Can you show us the evidence for this please?
- What are the actual statistics?
- If I go ahead with your recommendations, what limits does this place on my labour? Will I be ruled out of the MLU, for example?
- Why do you feel this is necessary at this point?

- What are the side effects for the baby?
- I'm hearing that you are not very supportive of my preferences. Can you recommend another doctor/midwife who would be?

All non-urgent discussions should end with time to think. You can say, 'Can you give us some privacy to discuss this?' or 'I will be in touch with my decision as soon as possible.'

*Georgie's Story*

*Georgie attended an extra appointment for a scan at her local hospital. She had been told she had low Papp A (low levels of a protein made by the placenta, which may or may not affect the size and growth of the baby). Georgie had been tested for this protein without consent and so had been unaware that it could affect her pregnancy and birth options. During her appointment, the consultant obstetrician spoke to her regarding the test results by saying 'Because you have low Papp A, we won't let you go past 40 weeks, so I will book you for an induction,' and then asked Georgie and her partner 'how do you feel about that?' There was no conversation about why, or what the risks and benefits are to having low Papp A, having an induction, or remaining pregnant past 40 weeks. Luckily, Georgie and her partner were well informed and told the doctor that they were not going to consent to the induction and didn't want to discuss it further. The obstetrician shocked them by immediately backing down and saying, 'no problem, that's fine,' and went on to agree that it was her body, and her choice. It was a complete turnaround from the conversation they had at the start of the consultation. Had Georgie not been previously made aware that she could say NO to the induction, or any other interventions offered to her, a date would have been scheduled and she would have been exposed to a procedure that carries multiple risks that had not been explained to her. Georgie went on to have a beautiful home water birth, giving birth to her son on his due date.*

---

### Dogma

**Dogma** (noun): *Something held as an established opinion. A fixed belief or set of beliefs that people are expected to accept without argument or doubt.*

There are so many myths relating to childbirth that need busting. Many of these myths have become embedded into the stories shared with pregnant women by doctors, midwives, family, and friends. In my experience, myths usually are spread without any evidence to back up the words or theories that are spoken of. They are simply thought of as true and factual. Whilst I don't profess to be an expert in evidence-based medicine myself, I read a lot and regularly signpost my clients to those that are. Dr Sara Wickham in the UK, Dr Rachel Reed in Australia, and Evidence Based Birth in the US are just three of the authors, bloggers, and podcasters that provide us with regular information that reviews evidence and dispel myths and dogma around the subject of maternity care. Don't let anyone tease you about seeking information online, as it can be more up to date and reliable there than much of what is shared with you by many medical professionals. Social media can be an excellent resource to help you find interesting quotes and statistics that validate your own philosophies about birth and support your decisions. Once you know your rights, you will feel more confident in speaking up.

## Classic Dogma Statements

- **Homebirth is dangerous.** No, it's not! There are plenty of studies to show that homebirth is as safe, if not safer, for most women who do not have an underlying health condition.

- **If you have gestational diabetes, you should be induced at 39 weeks.** Nope! If you are controlling your Gestational Diabetes Mellitus (GDM), your baby is not at any greater risk of being too big to fit through your pelvis.

- **Your placenta will stop working after you reach full term.** No, it won't! There is absolutely no evidence to support this at all. Your placenta does not have an expiration date! Just like all of the baby's other organs, it functions well to keep them alive until it is no longer needed.

- **If you are tired in labour, you won't have enough energy to push your baby out.** Ridiculous! During a physiological birth, you will always have the energy to push, because it's an uncontrollable instinct. Your body wakes you up with a huge surge of adrenaline and ideally the fetal ejection reflex will kick in and support you (see Chapter 6).

- **We always do delayed cord clamping.** This is not true! Many babies have their umbilical cord clamped and cut almost immediately at birth and are left without their full blood volume. Delayed is not the same as optimal, but even a delay is not happening in most hospitals.

- **It's against the law to decline care in pregnancy (wild pregnancy) and/or to give birth without medical assistance (freebirth).** Absolutely not true! It is completely legal in the UK to be pregnant and not access any medical care, although it is best to inform your GP that you are expecting so it does not look like you are trying to conceal the pregnancy. It is also perfectly legal to give birth without a midwife or doctor present, as long as whoever is in attendance with you is not acting as a medical professional. You do have a legal obligation to notify the chief administrative medical officer of the Health Board in your area of the birth within 36 hours, so it's important to find out any relevant information in advance and be clear on who you need to contact and how.

## Going Against Medical Advice

This chapter focusses on you learning to fully understand your rights in order to make decisions about your body and what is put into it or done to it. You also know that fear-based medicine is practiced out of fear of litigation, so recommendations are likely to be made to you in order to avoid the unpredictable, with a live baby at the end being the main goal. I am sure it's a relief to know that your care givers don't want anything bad to happen to your baby, but remember that the well-meaning doctor or midwife who cares for you on any given day or shift, does not have a greater interest in the health and well-being of your baby than you. Any repercussions from the decisions made about your care are yours to live with, not theirs. If you choose to decline advice given to you, it should be based on instinct, research, and respectful discussion. If that is not your experience, then you can politely ask for another practitioner to support you. If you struggle to vocalise your thoughts clearly, write them down ahead of time on paper or on your phone, as this can help you confidently express yourself. If you find the person speaking to you is using coercive language, then it is ok to tell them that you believe they are breaking the law. You can remind them that they need your consent to proceed, and you do not feel well informed. Try to always remain calm and respectful if possible.

## Medical Gaslighting

Medical gaslighting can happen when a care provider wrongly blames or inappropriately denies the patient (or pregnant woman) their reality in an attempt to invalidate them, dismiss them or convince them to accept recommendations.

Here are some examples.

- Your concerns about symptoms or sensations that don't feel right to you are dismissed.

- You are told you 'have to have' a particular test or procedure that you don't want.
- You are being scared into accepting an intervention by tactics that undermine your instincts, your research, your knowledge of your body, and your preferences.
- Your body is blamed for anything you experience in labour, or you are told that you didn't do enough to help yourself.

In any of these situations, I recommend you and your birth partner end the meeting immediately; tell your care provider their behaviour is unacceptable; speak to a more senior member of staff on shift; seek a second opinion; and/ or make a formal complaint.

If you choose not to accept what you are told despite being led to doubt your own body and instincts, you may have to be really direct, particularly in labour, and say something like:

- You are not listening to me.
- If anything happens to my baby, I will hold you personally responsible.
- Would you like to repeat what you have just said, so I can record the conversation?
- I want you to listen to my concerns or I will have to make a complaint against you.
- That is not respectful of my right to informed decision making.

- Kindly just document my preferences. I am declining at this time, not refusing care altogether.
- You are disrupting my labour, and I want you to leave.
- I do not consent—please leave.
- Anything you say to me from this point on I will consider harassment.

## Stockholm Syndrome

During your birth, depending on how long you are in labour, there may be several shift changes, and staff will come and go. Some you will like and connect with, whilst others you may not. If you have been fortunate to meet any of these people in advance, you may have a clear idea whether their personality is a good fit for you. It's hard to know what you need from someone who looks after you until you are in any given situation, and most of the time for a physiological birth, you need someone quiet and confident who just leaves you to it. I have, however, personally witnessed times during labour where some 'tough love' was needed, and a firm instruction given to motivate an exhausted client to keep going. What is important is that whenever someone speaks to you in labour, you feel safe and supported by them, and at no time should you feel scared and fearful. Stockholm syndrome—where you develop a coping mechanism to befriend your care provider in an attempt to prevent them from harming you—is becoming increasingly more common with women who admit to having a traumatic birth experience. Many couples are unaware that they can change their care provider and ask for a replacement. Whilst I can appreciate that it might not be easy to ask someone to leave your birth room, or approach the shift manager and request an alternative person looks after you, this is far better than finding yourself experiencing post-traumatic stress disorder (PTSD) in the postnatal period because you were cared for by someone who was unkind and made you feel unsafe.

## *Summary*

- **Consent is everything.** Nothing can be done or given to you without your consent. Whilst your care provider knows this, they might not always behave in a way that shows they do. It is important for you to only accept recommendations or procedures that you feel you have fully consented to. It is not uncommon for coercive comments to be made to convince you to agree to a particular procedure. Doctors and midwives are well known for suggesting you will be putting your child at risk of harm or death if you do not agree to their recommendations, or that you cannot receive care or adequate pain relief if you don't consent/agree to a vaginal examination. This is actually illegal, and you can remind them of this if necessary.
- **Decisions should be well informed.** It is impossible to make solid decisions about your care when you are not given information that spells out risks, benefits and alternatives to interventions or procedures offered. Finding

the courage to stand up for yourself and ask questions regarding your options might not always feel necessary. Only you will know if there is good reason to continue the conversation until you feel happy that you have all the information required when a decision needs to be made. If, however, during an antenatal appointment or your labour you are involved in a conversation with a care provider and you feel that you have not been given adequate details about their recommendations, then you will have to ask questions yourself to ensure you can make appropriate decisions.

- **Understand Relative vs Absolute Risk.** Most doctors and midwives make recommendations based on personal opinion or hospital guidelines, and not all are evidence-based. If you find yourself in a conversation with a care provider, either in pregnancy or during labour, and you are told there is a risk to you or your baby and an intervention is recommended, information should be shared with you to support your understanding of what those risks are. Rather than saying phrases like 'increased risk' or 'at a greater risk of,' they should give you statistics that help you to understand the absolute risk and look at more personalised information, giving you solid reasons for why they might be recommending a particular intervention. This will help you to decide which risk is greater: accepting the intervention, or not. All risks are yours to take.

# CHAPTER SIX
## Trust Your Body

*When the body is in charge, very little will go wrong.*

The human body is perfectly made to procreate, and nature designed every element of our being to help us not only survive but thrive as a species. Now that you are pregnant, there should be very little you need to do to prepare for birth, other than stay healthy and hydrated, because your body will lead the way. I know it's not that simple for everyone and learning to trust your body can take time. You may have had quite a journey to get to this point already, perhaps with a previous difficult birth experience where you felt your body let you down, a pregnancy loss, IVF, or other reasons you might feel sceptical about your body's capabilities, affecting your relationship with it. This is completely understandable, and I know many of you will be feeling this way, but one thing is for certain: regardless of how, your baby will be born, and I want you to make it the best experience for you. Through learning to trust your amazing body and its incredible capabilities, you can influence and shape the outcome of your birth.

## Learning to Trust Your Body

We have roughly 60,000 thoughts a day, and many of those are not positive or kind when they relate to ourselves. In order to learn to put complete trust in your body's ability to give birth to your baby in the way nature designed, you need to switch off the negativity and start focusing on ensuring your thoughts align with your plans. The words that we speak on this journey dictate everything, so you have to believe in the end of the story. See yourself after giving birth holding your baby in your arms. Picture the look on your face as you bask in the wonderful, proud feeling. If you align all your thoughts, words, and actions towards your dream birth, it's more likely to happen. Keep reminding yourself that your body is made to give birth to your baby! No matter what challenges you face, the deep-seated belief you have in your capability to give birth the way you are planning will support you to succeed. Practice the tools outlined in Chapter 3 to re-frame the neural pathways in your brain and remind yourself with daily affirmations that you trust your body completely. Any words spoken from someone who shows doubt in your ability will then bounce off you, because they cannot dampen this certainty.

## A Word About Dementors

In the popular Harry Potter books, Dementor is a name given to beings who steal happiness. They deprive human minds of intelligence and confidence, and they glory in despair. This is the name I give to all the people in life that show doubt in me. We all have them; they undermine our plans and belittle us for our choices. These are the people you ideally need to avoid as much as possible during your pregnancy. Do you already know who yours are? The ones whose advice you don't trust and with whom you should avoid sharing information about your birth plans because they will doubt you or your ability to give birth in the way you know you are capable of. Don't give them any power when it comes to your thoughts and plans. Dementors can walk away with your perfect birth experience, so make sure that doesn't happen to you.

### Due Dates are Nonsense

When you are first aware you are pregnant, it's easy to work out your estimated due date (EDD) based on your last menstrual period. There are so many online calculators that take the date you input and add 280 days. These tools make the assumption that we all gestate for the same length of time based on Naegele's rule. Fritz Naegele was a German hospital administrator who used the bible and hospital data in the 1800s to determine the normal length of pregnancy. Naegele's rule assumed that every woman ovulates on day 14 of their cycle, which of course we now know is not the case. The reality is that only 5% of pregnant women give birth on their actual date.

In addition, when you calculate this so-called due date, it adds on two weeks that you were not even pregnant; the date you conceived is calculated from the first day of your last menstrual period, around two weeks before ovulation. So, unlike putting a date in the diary for a wedding or event where the date is set in stone, it's best to think that you have a 'due month' or 'due window.' A guide, a rough idea, an approximate time that you can prepare for the baby's arrival, but with a degree of flexibility. Ideally, it's best to also tell friends and family a date that is a few weeks beyond the one you were given. If/when that date comes and goes, there will be less pressure on you overall to go into labour. Every day in late pregnancy genuinely feels like a lifetime for most women. You feel pressure in all directions, not only from yourself, but from your partner who is on call and scared to go anywhere, and who treats you like a ticking time bomb who could go off at any moment. Try to eliminate any additional stresses by remembering that due dates are nonsense, and take the approach that your baby will come in their own time. By adding a couple of weeks onto the end of the official EDD, you won't have to listen to well-meaning family and friends constantly checking in to ask, 'Have you had that baby yet?' The word 'late' won't exist, because the baby is not late. Your baby doesn't know there is a clock; they will just continue to grow and develop until they are ready to release the hormones that start labour.

## Never Chase Your Labour

Pregnant women are encouraged by books, articles, well-meaning family members, friends, doctors and midwives to believe that they should encourage labour to start with the use of certain foods and treatments, sex, or long walks. Worse, they accept methods of medical induction—which include 'stretch and sweeps'—long before their baby is ready to be born. Your care providers should be leaving you alone and not intervening in a perfectly designed system. You should not be subjected to interventions which can leave you incapable of giving birth physiologically to a baby that you have grown beautifully to this point. By trusting your body and your instincts deeply, you can confidently decline all offers of interference and let your baby decide when to come. With no external pressures or expectations regarding date and gestation, your mind will be clear, oxytocin can build, and your baby will find the right position and trigger labour at the perfect moment for them. This ensures that their lungs are mature and ready for the outside world, they will release essential hormones that help prepare them for labour, they will have had more time to align into the right position and will be exposed to vital microbes that greet them on arrival and begin building their immune system. So, if you want to eat certain foods, have relaxing treatments, take holistic remedies, have lots of sex, and go on long walks, do so because they are pleasurable and make you feel relaxed and happy, not because you are trying to evict your baby before their true birthday.

## Signs of Labour

In the last weeks of pregnancy, as your hormones start to change, you may notice signs that you are preparing for birth. Some women show an abundance of energy and 'nest' by cleaning and clearing to make space for the new baby. Others start to instinctively wrap themselves up in a protective bubble and withdraw from the world, preparing to 'go inwards.' The main thing is to just go with the flow. Lean into this time and try not to overthink it. Read a book, go to the cinema, a museum or gallery, plan a dinner party etc:- This is a time for enjoyment and oxytocin, so avoid stress or arguments where possible.

### Mucus Plug and Bloody Show

One of the first signs of labour for some is the loss of your mucus plug or to see it mixed with blood (called a 'bloody show'). The two are slightly different but can often occur at the same time. The loss of the mucus plug can happen as early as a week or more before labour begins, whereas the bloody show is a clearer sign that the cervix is working well to prepare for birth and is streaked or tinged with blood. For some women it is a slight pink tinge, and for others it can be really 'bloody' and they are concerned they are bleeding. If you were bleeding, it would be obvious, as bright red blood would be runny and soak a pad. I recommend that you become familiar with images of a bloody show, which you typically discover when you wipe after going to the toilet. I have had many clients' birth plans sabotaged because they were experiencing normal physiological signs of labour, but because there was more blood than they were expecting, they wanted reassurance. Whenever you call the hospital to ask a question in this scenario, you will be advised to go in and be checked out 'just in case.' This can sadly lead to a birth becoming medically managed unnecessarily, so take great care and follow your instincts.

*Please note: Sex can also cause a bloody discharge at this time in pregnancy.*

## Contractions

As your cervix (the neck of the womb) begins to soften, thin out and open, you will start to feel contractions (often referred to as 'surges,' 'rushes,' 'tightenings,' or 'waves'). Your body is working hard to draw your cervix upwards and out of the way for the baby to pass through. There are many magical changes happening inside, so it is incredibly important to rest as much as possible during this time. There should be no rush, no time limit, no pressure! You can expect your contractions to be inconsistent initially, often with no real pattern. As your oxytocin rises, they will become more regular and noticeably increase in length.

### Turning Contractions

Your clever body knows when your baby is not yet lined up in your pelvis and it helps them to turn from a posterior position, where the baby's head and back is near your spine, to an anterior one where the baby's spine is closer to the front. As your baby descends through the pelvis, your contractions will be working hard to encourage them to rotate, so you may experience what I call 'turning contractions.' These tend to be longer than regular contractions and may last up to 1.5 to 2 minutes, sometimes coming in clusters. A classic sign you are experiencing these longer contractions is that you have powerful sensations early on in labour, but they are inconsistent. Sometimes your labour stops and starts. The best way to manage this time is by adopting a forward-leaning position, keeping the baby off your spine where possible, and resting and 'flopping' (relaxing your entire body) between every contraction. Soften your jaw and shoulders, let go of all tension, close your eyes and trust in your body. You'll find that if you can breathe through this phase, your baby will move, so the back of their head will then press on your cervix more evenly, which helps it to open. Your contractions should then slow down, shorten and regularise, giving you a good break between. It's helpful to remind yourself that your body is clever and knows how to turn your baby during this time.

Websites like **spinningbabies.com** can show you and your partner positions to adopt that encourage the baby to move. I recommend the side-lying release and forward-leaning inversion. You can visit the website and practice these positions in advance of your birth, to familiarise yourselves with the concepts, and then, if necessary, refer back to this on the day if you need to.

### Waters Breaking

Around 10% of women will experience their waters releasing as the first sign of labour. This happens when the membranes around the baby that contain the amniotic fluid break, and the fluid either trickles out in a steady flow, or gushes out following a 'pop.' You'll know it's the waters breaking when liquid continues to leak out for the duration of labour and birth. If you suspect your waters have broken, put on a sanitary pad, as each time the baby moves, the fluid usually continues leaking out. If leakage stops, it is more likely to be *cervical weeping*, where collagen fibres liquify and sometimes pool in the vagina and release. Cervical weeping does not affect your bag of waters, so no action needs to be taken.

For most women, around 70%, contractions will begin shortly after their waters break, usually within 24 hours. Whilst it is recommended that you contact your midwife or hospital to let them know what is happening, you should remember that if they offer you the opportunity to go to the hospital to confirm it was your waters, remember it is just that—an offer. Any journey you make at this point will be counterproductive to the release of oxytocin, so tune into your instincts and consider whether you are ok and your baby is ok. For instance, are your waters clear with no odour? If everything seems all right, you may want to stay at home and relax. If you decide you want to make that call, you can have a sensible discussion with the midwife on duty about what your options include, perhaps choosing to stay home for a while longer. If you do go in to be monitored, you may also be advised to have an examination or swab test using a speculum to confirm your waters have broken. Ideally vaginal examinations (VEs) and anything else entering the vagina should be kept to a minimum or declined completely at this stage, as they will increase your risk of infection. If you do decide to decline, you can inform your care provider that you prefer to just wait and observe the fluid. If it continues to leak, then it is a clear sign that it was in fact your waters. Sexual intercourse is also an infection risk and is not advised once your waters have broken. If labour doesn't begin within 24 to 48 hours, you will be told to report to the hospital for an induction of labour. This recommendation is entirely optional and based on the doctor's concern that you are at increased risk of infection, so ask them what the absolute risk of infection is.

Looking at an NHS information leaflet, I found the following:

> After your waters have released there is a small increase in the chance that you and your baby could develop an infection. Before the waters release there is a 1 in 200 chance of infection and after they release (and within the first 24 hours) this increases to 1 in 100. At each 24 hours after this the chance doubles, so at 48 hours the chance is 2 in 100 and at 72 hours it is 4 in 100.

If you turn the risk around, that means 99% of women after 1 day will not have developed an infection, 98% after 2 days and 96% after 3 days. If you decide to follow your body and let labour begin in its own time, you can check your temperature regularly, avoid all vaginal examinations, observe the colour and smell of your amniotic fluid, and keep a record of your baby's movements. Your care providers should support your decision.

***Please note:*** *If your waters have been broken for longer than 24 hours, and you give birth in a hospital environment rather than at home or MLU, paediatricians within that unit may want to give your baby antibiotics 'just-in-case.' This action is not risk free and can have long-term side effects for your child. You should discuss this eventuality with your care providers when deciding on a plan.*

## Meconium

The presence of meconium (baby's first poo) in the amniotic fluid will be noticeable because your waters will not be clear. Old meconium, often called insignificant, can be a yellow or green colour. It typically signifies that the baby opened its bowels before labour began and is usually not serious; it can simply indicate that the baby's digestive system has reached maturity. Fresh meconium, on the other hand, is thick, black, and sticky, and if present during labour, is thought to be an indication that the baby isn't coping and a sign of distress. I recommend you do your research in advance of labour and look at images of both. In the event that meconium is present, you will then instinctively know if you want to decline or accept interventions like continuous fetal monitoring in an obstetric unit.

## Plan for the Long Haul

If labour is long, it can be easy for anyone to lose focus. Fatigue and exasperation can diminish hormone production, and this is where doubt creeps in. You might be experiencing prodromal labour, where you have contractions that come and go over several days. They start and stop, often subsiding in the morning and picking up again at night when it's quiet and dark. Contractions can be regular and long, and yet have no effect on labour progress. Or, you might have a longer latent phase, the time when your cervix is softening and thinning and you may have contractions, which can take hours or days. For some women labour is lengthy, especially a first labour, so it's important to plan and prepare for that. No one has a crystal ball to determine how fast or slow your labour will be, so planning for a longer labour makes it easier, helping you to go the distance if long labour becomes a reality for you

In preparation for a longer labour I recommend the following:

**Don't wake your partner or ask them to come home from work at the first sign of labour.** If contractions start in the daytime, then get comfortable; you are producing enough oxytocin for labour to be triggered, so keep doing whatever you're doing and rest as much as possible. If you feel contractions begin overnight, you are also clearly producing enough oxytocin, so stay where you are and sleep in between contractions. If it stops by the morning, you will have wasted little to no energy. If it continues, you are obviously in labour and can carry on resting until you are ready to move into a different position.

**Eat regular meals and snacks and drink plenty of water to stay hydrated.** Ensure that you are giving your body plenty of fuel for your labour.

**Avoid engaging with your maternity care provider for as long as possible,** unless you have a concern about yourself or your baby. Once you engage with any medical professional in early labour, your personalised clock starts ticking. You now have a time limit placed on you of how quickly your care provider believes you should be progressing. Any phone conversations you have, or questions you ask regarding your circumstances will be documented and can give evidence of the need for intervention if your progress is not meeting their expectations. If you instinctively feel that things are ok with you and the baby, then try to avoid contact until it becomes necessary and you are ready for support, unless you are receiving care from an Independent Midwife, birth keeper, or doula.

**Don't communicate with friends and family or on social media.** The minute you tell others that you think you might be in labour, a whole other pressure starts to take effect. People ask you questions and want to give advice; their fears kick in, and if labour is long, they will worry—and no doubt worry you, landing you in the amber zone where progress is slow.

## Lisa's Story

*Lisa's first baby was born by caesarean section after her labour was deemed to be 'not progressing' by her care providers. She hired me as her doula when she was expecting her 2nd baby, and we spoke in detail about what she wanted to achieve this time around. During our first antenatal appointment, Lisa shared that she would be giving birth at home because she didn't want to feel under pressure to perform in a certain time frame, which she knew could lead to her birth being 'meddled with' before her body or baby were ready. She made the decision not to tell her family. She felt that they would feel scared about her plan to home birth, and so she kept it to herself. As labour established, her living room was dark and cosy and she was definitely in the zone. Her sounds were low, and I sat in the corner quietly out of her eyeline. For a long time, I wasn't sure she knew I was there. As the surges intensified, Lisa would lift her right leg onto the edge of the sofa and lunge. I witnessed her opening her pelvis about 7 or 8 times. When we talked after the birth, I discovered she had no memory of those instinctive movements whatsoever. During our postnatal visit a week later, we spoke about how she had tuned into her body and clearly created space on the right side without ever needing to think about it. Her body knew exactly what to do to get her baby out because she was left to birth in complete freedom. No noise, questions, or bright lights to distract her. It was perfect.*

## Making Sounds with Confidence

It is perfectly instinctive and normal to make raw, guttural, and often loud sounds during labour. To squash these sounds is inadvisable if they are coming from a place deep within you. They are helpful to the process and support your dilation. Make whatever sounds you feel like with confidence, and don't feel embarrassed. My only warning is that it is usually unhelpful to make sounds that go upwards in pitch, like a scream. These sounds don't release tension, they increase it, and they are counterproductive. Tell your birth partner that if they hear you making high-pitched sounds, they should remind you to soften your jaw, relax your shoulders, and send your sounds downwards, keeping the tones low.

## Resting Between Contractions

During labour your body is working hard, and you can get tired very quickly. It is important to recognise the need to rest and relax between contractions from as early in the process as possible. By finding comfortable positions that facilitate your ability to soften all your muscles and flop into a deeply relaxed state, you will be able to sustain labour for as long as it takes. The precious breaks that you have after the contractions end should be used as a time to switch off your thoughts, conserve your energy and replenish yourself with water and snacks when necessary.

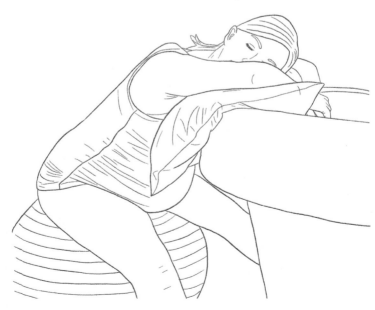

## Ways to Assess Progress

In days gone by, there were no machines or technical ways to assess progress of labour. So, midwives just observed! They spent time noticing women's behaviour to see if there were repetitive patterns, sounds, or physical symptoms—and they witnessed many. Women across the world behave the same in labour, make the same noises and perform similar actions. When left to their own devices, women often adopt positions that facilitate as much room in their pelvis as possible, staying upright and gravity assisted.

Here are other ways that your progress can be noted:

- You have to continue focusing on your breath even after the contraction has ended.
- You start to go inwards and communicate less.
- The temperature of your feet, ankles, and lower legs can become colder.
- A congestion line may appear that runs from your anus up to the top of your butt crack.
- You might show transitional behaviour, where you begin to wake up and become a little wild and present: a clear sign of adrenaline.
- You might vomit, which can be a sign of pressure and signify that you are progressing.
- You might release whatever poo is left in your rectum. When this poo is pushed out, it means the baby's head is near.

## Your Cervix and Your Throat

Your cervix, located between the vaginal canal and the womb (uterus), can change in a multitude of ways during labour and birth. It expands and stretches like no other organ, and then returns to its normal size within hours after your baby is born. Your throat is directly linked to your cervix by the vagus nerve and is deeply connected to your emotions and how you think and feel. Both can be affected by stress levels, breathing patterns, and sounds. When one is tight, usually so is the other. For this reason, it's important to remember that your jaw in particular is very influential to your labour progress. If you are aware that you always clench this area, you are going to need to train yourself to remember to relax and soften your jaw, lips, and throat, or your cervix might remain tight too. As you progress into labour, remember to soften your mouth, make low sounds with confidence, moan, and breathe; these will all help your cervix to soften and open. I recommend you follow Emma, @thenakeddoula, on Instagram, who calls this 'Floppy face, Floppy fanny.' Emma is a visual illustrator who uses images of 'Miss Fanny' and others to show you how to trust your body and own your birth experience.

## The Fear-Tension-Pain Cycle

It's not uncommon for women to fear the pain of labour, because it is unknown. Sometimes it can become massively built up in our minds, and many women will write themselves off from the outset believing they won't be able to manage throughout labour. I think this helps them to prepare for disappointment. You might think or say things like 'I will never cope with labour' or believe your ability to cope has something to do with your pain threshold or stamina. Trust me, it doesn't! Dr Grantley Dick-Read, author of the book Childbirth Without Fear, performed a study in 1916, where women from poorer communities with little or no education were compared to women from more affluent backgrounds. He found that the poorer women had simple, easy births, whereas the better educated women cried out in agony. He determined the difference was all fear driven and developed his theory of the fear–tension–pain cycle. When we feel fear in the body, it is held within our tissues—in every fibre of our being. When we get stuck in a cycle of fear, it leads to tension in the body. This will inevitably cause you more pain. As fear creeps in, tension builds, and the fear-tension-pain cycle takes over.

## The Power of the Breath

Breathing is the most powerful way to manage sensations in the early stages of labour, and it is helpful for you to concentrate on your breath during this time, regardless of whether you go on to use other birth management methods. If you can distract yourself from any sensations you are feeling by using your breath as a focus, you will find it easier as labour progresses. This will help your endorphin and oxytocin levels to rise. In particular, you will benefit from using your outbreath to really relax and let go, as it is very hard to tense up on a long exhalation. As labour continues, you may have moments where you feel overwhelmed and forget to breathe altogether. This tightens the throat and therefore the cervix and introduces adrenaline. Ideally, you want your birth partner to step in before this happens and remind you to breathe, or possibly even breathe with you until you are back on track. It is important to speak to them in advance about what you would prefer them to do in that scenario and what to look out for. Signs that you are holding tension and beginning to struggle might include your shoulders rising, or your vocalisations becoming high pitched. If they see you losing control of your breath, ask them to stand close to you and quietly say something like: 'Use your breath' or 'Take a nice deep breath in and let this one go' or 'Would it help if I breathe with you?'

## Focused Breathing Techniques for Labour

In early labour, breathing in a focused way should feel easy as your contractions should hopefully be short and spaced out. I recommend slow breathing techniques like the following.

### Ujaii breath (ocean breath)

This is a classic yoga breath, which is very useful throughout labour and wonderful for the early days with a new baby, who will love hearing your calm, deep rhythmic breathing as you hold them close. Begin practicing this technique by sitting in a well-supported position. Take a deep inhalation in through the nose, and then breathe out through the mouth as if seeing your breath in front of you on a really cold day. The sound you make is a 'haaaaa' sound, which is soft like a whisper. Breathe this way a few more times, and then as you become more confident, progress to leaving the mouth closed on the exhale. You should still be able to hear an audible sound at the back of your throat (described as sounding like the ocean). Ujaii breath encourages focus and concentration, whilst also bringing a sense of calm as the belly rises on the inhale and falls on the exhale.

### Counting breath

Establish a deep, rhythmic breath, and then silently begin to count the inhale and exhale: Breathing in 1 2 3 4 / Breathing out 1 2 3 4 5 6. The numbers you count don't matter, but the exhale should be longer than the inhale. Even though your mind may wander off many times, keep bringing your attention back to the counting and away from any sensations that you are feeling.

### Let go breath

Again, once a lovely deep breathing pattern is established, you can begin to inhale and then silently think the word Let, and then as you exhale, you think the word Go. Each time, you can scan down the body from the top of the head to the tips of the toes, softening and relaxing so there is no tension at all.

### Golden thread breath

With this breathing technique, you will breathe out through the mouth. Take a deep breath in through the nose to begin, and as you exhale, breathe out a fine stream of air through a small gap that you create between your top lip and bottom lip. As you exhale, you can imagine the fine stream of air as a thin golden thread that carries your attention out into the distance. The purpose of this breath is to slow down the exhalation, which can help to distract the mind. As you breathe and your thoughts travel further and further away from you, you can get lost in the focus. It is described by many women as a useful breathing technique for early labour.

### Dandelion breath

As the surges intensify, you might find that you are more inclined to want to breathe out of your mouth as you exhale, more and more. In this instance, the breath that I find the most successful is one I call dandelion breath. This is a powerful breathing technique that provides you with strength and focus. It is also the reason I chose a dandelion symbol for my books and my brand overall; a dandelion can thrive in difficult conditions and has the ability to rise above challenges, a perfect analogy for a woman in labour. To try it, imagine a fluffy-headed dandelion. Take a deep breath in and as you exhale, purse the lips and breathe out fully through the mouth. Your breath should flow out in a steady stream as if blowing towards the dandelion and scattering the seeds far and wide. Each time you exhale, you notice at the end that there is a natural pause. Wait until this is over before taking another long deep breath in, and then breathe out forcefully, as if you are trying to make a gust of wind.

## The Female Pelvis

It's hard to describe just how amazing the female pelvis is in a book, so hopefully your antenatal course will help you to feel familiar with this incredible bony structure that your baby navigates during the birth process. The female pelvis, wider than the male equivalent, comes in a variety of differing shapes. In medical school, doctors and midwives are taught about the four most widely recognised. Of those, over 50% of Caucasian women have a Gynecoid pelvis, while nearly half of women of African descent have an Anthropoid shape. About 25% of all women have an Android pelvis, and only 5% are said to have a Platypelloid pelvis. During pregnancy, the hormone relaxin enables the pelvis to become more mobile, thereby softening the ligaments and joints in preparation. As labour begins, and the baby moves down, regardless of what shape pelvis you have, the soft bones in the baby's head will mould to fit the space. At the top of your pelvis (known as the brim or inlet) where the baby first begins to descend, it is widest from left to right or hip to hip. Once the baby's head is in the pelvic cavity (or mid-pelvis), it needs to rotate around in order for their shoulders to have enough room to drop in. This lines up the head with the outlet, which is widest from front to back. The baby will usually then turn again to birth the shoulders, like a key turning in a lock. It's helpful if you can adopt an upright or side-lying position during this time, so that your sacrum (triangular bone at the base of the spine) and coccyx (tailbone) then have the ability to lift and move out of the way. This enables your pelvis to open by as much as 30%.

## Rhombus de Michaelis

During the process of pushing your baby out, the triangular bone at the base of your spine (the sacrum) has the capability to move. Your lower back literally lifts and opens to create more space. The kite-shaped area just below your waist is called the 'Rhombus de Michaelis.' If at the time of pushing, your baby still needs to turn, this lifting will help to maximise any extra space required, so ideally an upright and forward position can facilitate descent and rotation of the baby. Interestingly, some women lift their arms upwards at this time, in order to feel stable and secure. The more space your body can create the better, so always remember to follow your instincts and move into positions that feel right for you.

## Sphincter Law

If you feel unsafe or unsettled during labour, your cervix has the potential to 'un-dilate,' its opening shrinking in size. If you experience a change in your circumstances, or a different care provider comes on shift whom you dislike, your labour can be dramatically affected. For many women the reduction in cervical dilation occurs during a VE (vaginal exam). In the book *Ina May's Guide to Childbirth,* midwife Ina May Gaskin talks about 'sphincter law.' She explains that some women may have progressed to a certain stage in labour, and when a VE takes place, the cervix shrinks back away from the fingers, because it doesn't like to be poked and prodded. Midwife and author Sara Wickham calls this same phenomenon 'cervical recoil.' A common story at my pregnancy yoga class involves a woman and her birth partner leaving for hospital, believing the labour to be advanced. During a vaginal examination she is found to be 3–4 cm dilated, and though she's a little disappointed, she is advanced enough to remain in hospital and not be sent home. Within an hour or two, the woman shows signs that she is feeling an urge to push and no one believes her. In this instance, I suspect that she was more likely to have been 6 or 7 cm dilated upon arrival at the hospital, and her cervix simply closed down when the examination was performed—returning back to where it had been shortly afterwards.

*Emily's Story*

*Emily had a VE and was found to be 6 cm dilated at 4 pm in the afternoon after a reasonably long labour so far. She was progressing nicely now and was feeling relaxed and confident that all was going well. At 8 pm she was examined again, just before her midwife went off shift, and was fully dilated. She had no urge to push, so Emily just kept breathing through her contractions, but the new midwife who had entered the room was keen to get things going. She asked Emily many questions over the next hour: 'Do you feel anything?' 'Have you got any pressure in your bottom?' 'Want to try having a push with the next contraction?' Emily was under huge pressure to perform and was inwardly feeling annoyed at the new midwife. After a few hours the midwife asked to assess Emily again and found her to be 5 cm dilated. The midwife blamed the first midwife for making a mistake and informing Emily that she was fully dilated when she clearly wasn't. In my opinion, Emily's cervix had decreased from 10 cm to 5 cm because of all the questions and the pressure to perform. In the end Emily didn't progress any further and had an abdominal birth. It was so frustrating for her. I believe that if she had asked for a different midwife and had been able to relax and feel safe again, her cervix would have returned to being fully dilated and her baby would have been born without the need for surgery.*

## Rest and Be Thankful

At the end of the dilation phase of labour, it is common for contractions to slow down and the gaps between them to become wider. This is a physiological event and one that you can trust as being completely normal. The late natural birth advocate and author Sheila Kitzinger calls this the 'rest and be thankful' stage. A period of time that can occur between dilation and pushing, when there is a temporary lull and contractions slow down or stop altogether. You may fall asleep and really benefit from the break. At this stage, midwives often fear the labour may have stalled, when in fact it is simply the body's way of giving the uterus a moment to gather itself before going in for the big push. If you notice your contractions start to space out, or tail off for a period of time, rest down and relax, enjoying the respite. You need to switch off your brain and let go of any tension in your body. Your uterus knows exactly what it is doing by taking this short break, and it will soon kick back into action again.

**Please note:** *If at any time during an obvious 'rest and be thankful' stage, the midwife or doctor suggests a synthetic oxytocin drip to bring back the contractions, I recommend you request an hour to rest first. In my experience, the wait usually does the trick and the contractions come back on their own.*

## Pushing for Primips

I always loved the article written by Canadian midwife/ birth attendant Gloria Lemay, called 'Pushing for Primips.' I have shared this so many times with clients over the years, and it has been incredibly useful in helping them understand the pushing phase and how to manage it for the first time. Give it a read at **wisewomanwayofbirth.com** (see the Resources section at the back of the book). In the article, Gloria talks of the need for patience when a woman is pushing out her first baby (primip). She describes the process as 'a space in time where her obstetrical future often gets decided.' She explains that much mischief can take place when a woman feels pressure to perform and begins to push before she is ready. This is a very delicate stage, and she cautions that a vaginal examination at this point can cause a delay in the process. This opinion goes against the medical narrative that a woman should not push until she is found to be fully dilated or she may cause herself harm. If the cervix were to swell, the baby would struggle to be born vaginally. I suspect that if a midwife or doctor has ever discovered a woman with a swollen cervix, it is more likely that it was caused by directed pushing, and not the woman gently pushing instinctively. As Gloria goes on to explain, the final part of dilation and the early pushing stage are vitally important, and no woman ever swelled her own cervix by listening to her body. She speaks of the need for midwives to change their notion of what is happening in the pushing phase with a primip from 'descent of the head' to 'shaping of the head.' Each expulsive sensation shapes the head of the baby to conform to the contours of the mother's pelvis. This can take time and lots of patience.

## Need to Push vs Actual Pushing

If you start to feel an urge to push, then this is usually an obvious sign that you are nearly, but not quite ready to begin pushing—so just keep breathing. If you are experiencing a pushy sensation during each contraction, but only at the peak, then just follow your body and breathe. When you begin to push, it will be unmistakeable, and you won't be able to stop it. It's the same as if you were feeling the need to poo, but not actually pooing or feeling nauseous but not actually vomiting. Some women at this stage fall asleep during the longer gaps between contractions—a clear sign that your body is working hard but not quite awake enough for the expulsive pushes that will soon follow. I want you to avoid a situation where you suspect you are close, so you begin to push because you think you are ready. Sometimes the position of the baby's head may trigger a sensation prematurely, which may explain why you are feeling like the urge is there. These sensations are normal but remember there is a big difference between a sensation, and an overwhelming urge that you couldn't stop if you tried. When you are pushing, you should also feel very awake. No longer sleepy, but capable of anything, as your body has now entered fight or flight mode. If you understand the difference between feeling an urge to push, versus the sensation of being-unable-to-stop-it-if-you-tried actual pushing, you won't push until you are supposed to. The pressure will move from your belly to your rectum, and active pushing will begin with a feeling of needing to bear down. At this point, you won't have to tell anyone that you feel an urge to push, because they will hear it and see it for themselves.

## Fetal Ejection Reflex

The pushing phase is an extremely important part of the birthing process, and it can be easy or hard, depending on your understanding of how involuntary that process is when it is completely physiological. By trusting that your body will tell you when the time is right, you will be able to work with an internal force that is designed to push the baby out—a mechanism a bit like projectile vomiting. French obstetrician and childbirth specialist Michel Odent speaks of a huge surge of adrenaline that the woman can experience at this exact point in labour, which wakes you up and helps to expel the baby quickly and efficiently. This is called the 'fetal ejection reflex.' Unlike vomiting, however, this reflex is pretty delicate, and the minute an outside influence arises and distracts you, this reflex and its benefits can be lost. Some women are more sensitive to their immediate environment than others at this stage. It is therefore important to expect this sensitivity, and anyone present should be incredibly mindful of remaining quiet and protective of your space during this time. This is not a good moment for you to be offered vaginal examinations, be asked questions, or be given suggestions, as it can delay you from feeling an overwhelming urge to push. Hopefully with the optimal environment, your body will do all the work itself and the baby will be born quickly and easily. Remember, you will be fully awake at this stage, and you will always have enough energy to push, despite feeling really sleepy only moments earlier.

**Please note:** *As adrenaline starts to flood your body, you may appear agitated or distressed. This can be a clear sign you are entering transition. It is normal at this point to want to use your safety word. Share this information with your birth partner so they can feel prepared for this moment and will be able to trust that your labour is progressing perfectly.*

## Tearing and Episiotomy

Your vaginal opening and perineum are capable of stretching beautifully to accommodate your baby's head and body during the final stages of labour. When birth is left to unfold in its own time, it's unlikely there will be any deep wounds or trauma to this area. Occasionally a woman might experience small skin tears or grazes—known as *first degree*—that will heal perfectly well on their own. If the baby's head position is slightly off centre or they are born with their hand by the side of their head, a deeper tear can occur, known as *second degree*. It is important to keep this area clean in the days following birth while it heals. You might feel a stinging sensation when you go to the toilet, so drink plenty of fluids to dilute your urine and stay hydrated. Deeper tears, known as *third* or *fourth degree,* can affect the muscle and will need to be sutured. Such tears are more likely to occur in non-physiological births. Since the overmedicalisation of childbirth, with women given medication and directions to push, deeper tears have become more common. Rarely, depending on the circumstances, a woman may be offered an episiotomy, where the doctor or midwife cuts the perineum in order to create more space for the baby's head to be born. This is more common in an assisted birth, such as one using forceps. If you are keen to avoid any deep tears or cuts to your genitals, be really clear to your care providers that you do not want anyone offering guidance during the pushing stage and you want to breathe slowly if you feel a stinging sensation, which is simply helping you know when the baby is coming. Try not to rush the process; just follow whatever your body is guiding you to do.

**Please note:** *Depending on where you give birth, your midwife or doctor might offer you the option to protect your perineum as your baby's head is crowning. This involves placing a cloth and their gloved hands directly in the area of your vagina and perineum to support and slow down descent of the baby's head. This once again brings medical management and possible side effects to the birthing process. Your viewpoint on whether to accept the offer might differ if you are offered perineal support during a physiological birth versus a managed one.*

## Delayed v Optimal Cord Clamping

Cutting and clamping the umbilical cord should not be anyone's priority in the immediate moments after birth. Ideally your baby should be left alone to transition from womb to world gently. At the point when the baby takes their first breath and the lungs inflate, the cord naturally begins to pulsate, ensuring any blood still in the placenta is pumped quickly into the baby. That remaining blood typically represents about 30% of their overall blood volume. At the same time, Wharton's jelly—which is inside the cord protecting the arteries and vein and is responsible for keeping the cord in a twisted shape—begins to liquefy. The cord then starts to unwind, becoming loose and limp by the time it is empty. Understanding the difference between *delayed cord clamping* and *optimal cord clamping* at this stage can make a big difference to your baby and the amount of blood volume they receive. Many hospitals and homebirth team midwives have delayed cord clamping as standard in their guidelines; this typically involves severing the cord after a couple of minutes. Optimal cord clamping in comparison, involves leaving the cord alone until it is white and empty and no longer of any benefit to the baby.

With optimal cord clamping, babies receive:

- 30% more iron-rich blood. It would take approximately 6 months to replenish this if lost at birth.
- More oxygen to the brain, which continues to be provided to them as their lungs transition.

- 60% more red blood cells that carry oxygen, giving your baby extra support.
- More white blood cells to help fight infections.
- More stem cells, which have the genetic potential to prevent and repair damage throughout the body.

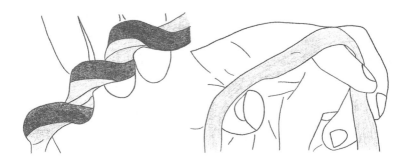

### Requesting Optimal Cord Clamping

If you request optimal cord clamping, it needs to be written clearly on your birth plan, and, at the time the baby is born, repeated by you and or your birth partner. Unless you are very clear, your baby's umbilical cord may be cut prematurely. If you and the baby are skin to skin and are both well and comfortable, then there is absolutely no benefit to touching the cord at all. If, however, you are not comfortable, or there is a reason why the baby needs to be removed from you, then a conversation can be had in that moment about whether the cord should be cut to separate you from the baby. Sometimes a cord is short and may initially prevent the baby from being lifted onto your chest; however, it should begin to lengthen as the cord unwinds. You can see the change before your very eyes, and when you physically touch the cord you can feel it pulsate. As the cord lengthens and empties, it starts to become very obviously white and limp, so you will know when it is finished. If for any reason a paediatrician is called to the room, you should ensure they understand that leaving the cord to pulsate is a strong preference and should be respected unless a dire emergency requires them to rush your baby to the special care baby unit (SCBU). In most cases, even if the baby requires some initial support to breathe, that can be done next to you with the cord remaining intact, as it will continue to provide the baby with valuable oxygen. Write this preference down in your birth plan and point it out to your caregivers.

## Gut Health: The Human Microbiome

During the end of pregnancy, essential microbes will migrate to your vagina in preparation for birth. As the baby passes through and is born, the first microbial colonization takes place, and the baby is 'seeded' with this powerful cocktail of bacteria that is perfectly designed to populate their gut and begin building their immune system. This process is essential for the health and well-being of the baby. Sadly, many babies miss out on this gift because they are born via an abdominal birth and are exposed to antibiotics both during and after, which wipe out all the friendly bacteria that was meant to protect them. If this happens to your baby, there are other ways they can receive microbes: from the placenta, umbilical cord, amniotic fluid, a parent's skin and mouth, breastmilk, siblings, and pets.

A healthy immune system is developed when the baby is exposed to bacteria from all of the above, and what could be better than the germs of its own parents. Be mindful of allowing anyone in the room who is not related to touch your baby, as this is such a crucial time to the development of their gut and immune system. I personally never touch a newborn baby when working in the role of a doula. The thousands of different organisms inside you and on your skin are essential to keeping the baby safe, as 70% of their immune system is built in these moments. This makes skin-to-skin contact so important for at least an hour after birth, and it should be continued for as long as possible.

***Please note:*** *If you want your care provider to weigh your baby, I would encourage your partner to carry the baby to and from the scales themselves. This helps to preserve the newborn microbiome as much as possible.*

## The Golden Hour

The period of time after your baby is born should be unhurried. Ideally, the baby will not be touched by anyone other than you and your partner, where possible, for at least an hour. As the baby lies on your chest, their temperature begins to regulate, as you are designed to be a human incubator: quite cleverly, if the baby cools down, you will warm up, and vice-versa. If you are choosing to breastfeed, the golden hour gives your baby the opportunity to find their own way to the breast in a calm and relaxed manner. Often the baby will find their own way to the breast if given time and patience. Skin-to-skin contact during the golden hour also enables important hormones to be released that are crucial for the bonding process. In some hospitals and MLUs, the midwife will place a large egg timer in the room to remind staff to leave the baby alone and remain skin to skin with its mother. This means they are not allowed to touch, move or weigh the baby during these precious moments. As oxytocin levels rise and adrenaline levels diminish, your placenta will begin to separate from the uterine wall. If adrenaline levels remain high, it can often take longer. Any pressure to get the placenta out before it is ready further diminishes oxytocin levels, leaving the uterus unable to contract. For this reason, its best to ask anyone who is providing you with care to remain outside the room whilst you enjoy your golden hour.

## Trust Your Body

Your amazing body is capable of stretching, moving, adapting, and changing in any way it needs to in order to facilitate the safe arrival of your newborn. We are designed to survive and thrive, and when left alone to get on with giving birth it typically happens smoothly and easily. When outside influence is removed and there is no questioning of the process, it can be quick and straightforward, driven by hormone production and your parasympathetic nervous system flowing blood to your uterus. Your instincts are working behind the scenes to keep you both safe, and it should become obvious if you feel something is not going well. When others interfere and ask you questions, it can throw labour out. This includes introducing interventions such as vaginal exams that undermine and meddle with the body. When your care providers lack trust in your body's ability to continue, they want analytical discussion. You may hear words like 'I think you need some help here; we don't think you are progressing,' or 'Would you like something to take that pain away?' or 'If these contractions continue like this, you are not going to have the energy to push.' Despite others' lack of trust in your body's ability to give birth to any baby that you grow inside you, you must not buy into their misgivings. Words can undermine you and lead to intervention. Instead, be really clear on what you can do to secure the maximum amount of the right hormones being produced at the right time. This will help ensure you are progressing at the correct rate for your body and your baby, and you can trust that your body is working effectively with no need for assessments or discussion. Prepare your birth partner to understand just how amazing your body is and why it is important to leave well alone.

As Ina May Gaskin always said, 'Men take it for granted that their sexual organs can greatly increase in size and then become small again without being ruined. If obstetricians (and women) could understand that women's genitals have similar abilities, episiotomy and laceration rates might go down overnight.'

## Summary

- **When the body is in charge, very little will go wrong.**
  Learning to trust your body involves you fully believing in the process of birth and remembering that physiology works best when left alone. Creating the right conditions that enable you to feel safe, warm, and comfortable ensures your hormones will flow optimally.

- **Due dates are nonsense.** Your EDD is a rough guide to when your baby will be born, and only 5% of babies are born on their actual due date. It's best to prepare friends and family by giving them a date in the future, in order to take the pressure off you in those last weeks, avoiding adrenaline and extra stress.

- **Follow your body.** Once you have learned to trust your body, you can then just follow its lead in labour. Wait for your baby to trigger the cocktail of hormones your body needs, rest and relax and never chase your labour, avoid assessments that disrupt the flow, only push when you have an overwhelming urge, and leave the umbilical cord to pulsate until it is white and empty.

# CHAPTER SEVEN
## Birth Plans

*If I don't know my options, I don't have any.*

To bring all 5 key principles together and support you in achieving your physiological birth, I recommend you consider writing a *birth plan*: a set of preferences you have decided upon that includes everything you want to convey to your birth partner and care providers. The power of a birth plan isn't the actual plan, it's the process of becoming educated about all your options and understanding WHY you would choose to accept or decline any interventions offered. This is your birth, not your care providers'; a birth plan lets you take ownership of the decisions you are making. This list is something you can discuss with your birth partner in detail to make sure the most important elements you want to achieve are clear. I have shared with you my birth plan checklist so that you can explore your priorities and how to achieve them. For example, if you are investigating the option of a water birth, and it becomes obvious that this is really important to you, then you might have to consider giving birth at home with an inflatable pool to guarantee you will have access to it. If that is not an option, choose a local hospital or MLU who regularly facilitates water birth, put it at the top of your birth plan, and ask if a pool room is available when you call to say that you are in labour and ready for support. When I make that call on behalf of my clients, I will even ask the midwife to begin filling the pool so it is ready when we arrive. You can ask any hospital for their most recent statistics to ensure you choose wisely. When your birth plan is completed, you will have a valuable tool to use on the day. It becomes the first point of reference if any initial decisions need to be made, so make sure that you only write down the items that are realistic and relevant to your chosen venue and are achievable by your care provider. The way the birth plan is worded, and the individual preferences it includes, will help ensure that your wishes are easily understood and respected where possible.

### Birth Plan Checklist

This checklist can serve as a discussion guide for you to go through with your birth partner.

### 1. Philosophy of Birth

What does your dream birth look like? What do you want to achieve? What do you both need to learn and read in order to understand how to achieve your dream birth? What classes do you need to sign up for to boost your understanding of the decisions you may be expected to make during labour and birth?

## 2. Hospital Guidelines and Policies

Where can you give birth in your area: at home, or with midwife- or obstetric-led care? What facilities are available to choose from in each of these locations? Do you understand the guidelines and policies at your local unit that may affect you? The NICE intrapartum guidelines may help you understand any recommendations given; see their website at **nice.org.uk**, or ask your midwife for information, as policies do vary. What are your views on student observation? Monitoring? VEs? Induction? Pain relief? C-section? Do you know the pros and the cons of each in order to make a well-informed decision? Will you be required to submit a personalised care plan if you want to go against your local hospital's guidelines?

## 3. Environment

What surroundings might affect you? Do you and your birth partner know how to adjust your environment during labour? What will you want to take with you that will make you feel more at ease? (This category can include preferences on music, positioning, props, smells, gadgets, snacks, or breathing techniques).

## 4. Plan B or C

Sometimes plans change. Ensure you understand what you would want to happen if you had to change course.

What is your Plan B or C? If you had to go to theatre, would your partner come with you? Do you know and understand what options you have if an abdominal birth becomes necessary? If the baby had to go to special care, who would go with the baby?

## 5. After Care/Umbilical Cord and Placenta

Do you want to be the first person to touch the baby? Do you want the baby placed straight onto your skin? Do you understand the choices that can be made about the umbilical cord? Do you want an injection to expel the placenta, or do you want the placenta to come away on its own? Do you know what checks will be done to you? Do you know what checks will be done to the baby? Do you know why Vitamin K is recommended?

## 6. Feeding Your Baby

The baby may want to feed within the first few hours after birth. Have you decided how you want to feed your baby? If you intend to breastfeed, are you aware of the support in your area? Do you understand supply and demand? Do you know how many times per day a newborn baby feeds? Do you know what a tongue tie is? Are you aware of the common issues mothers face when learning to breastfeed? Do you have information on how to hand express or use a breast pump?

### 7. Putting a Plan Together

Once you have considered the questions above, done any research required and attended a good quality antenatal course, you can begin to put your preferences down on paper. I recommend a simple list that can be read quickly and easily. Be specific and don't add information that is not relevant. Please keep flexibility in mind if you are giving birth in a hospital environment with a more medical approach.

## Hard and Soft Boundaries

You shouldn't have to have the mindset that you are preparing for a fight when accessing maternity care on your terms. If you live in the UK, the law is on your side, and you can choose to have your baby wherever and in whatever way you want, including freebirth (birth with no medical care). I realise this kind of access varies greatly across the world; however, as far as I am aware, the right to bodily autonomy is universal. You do not need permission to give birth physiologically, but you may need to be assertive. In order to avoid conflict or issues when you are trying to express your wishes, I recommend getting really clear on what your boundaries are. Whilst nothing can be set in stone, if you definitely would prefer to avoid specific elements of routine care, for example, a vaginal examination, then consider the question: is that a hard boundary or a soft one? Am I likely to change my mind, or am I certain that I do not want anyone to check my cervix? If that is a hard boundary for you, then you need to make this very clear and be consistent with your message. This is important so that you are not confusing your partner or care provider. Many of my clients are prepared to be flexible on some elements of their care and not others. Another example is induction of labour. I have clients who would rather have an abdominal birth if their plan to give birth physiologically becomes impossible, so a hard boundary for them is to avoid any form of oxytocin drip installed to bring on the labour and contract the uterus synthetically. One client was adamant that she did not want her baby placed on her immediately and would prefer the baby to be cleaned and dried first. Each one of us is different, and we can take responsibility for our own feelings and express them however we need to. If for any reason your care provider is not in agreement with decisions you are making, then you will need to change to someone who is more supportive. Sometimes that involves being firm and repetitive when it comes to relaying your wishes and boundaries. This is especially important if you are met with coercive comments in an attempt to encourage you to change your mind about any decisions you are making.

## Personalised Care Plan

If you would like to give birth in a particular way that is considered to be outside of hospital guidelines, contact the Head of Midwifery, Deputy Head of Midwifery or Consultant Midwife at the hospital where you are booked to arrange for a personalised care plan to be put in place for you. Your community midwife will be able to help you identify who you need to speak to, and arranging a meeting should be pretty straightforward. You may want to ask your birth partner to attend with you. You can expect the midwife who facilitates this meeting to help you both understand the risks and benefits of the type of birth you are hoping for, and they may present you with facts or statements that are evidence based. Hiring a doula to support you and contacting organisations like Birthrights and AIMS can be incredibly beneficial in this scenario. (See the Resources section at the back of this book.) Health professionals are simply not used to women advocating for themselves, so initially they can take a strong approach by wanting to stick to the guidelines. But when you are consistent with your message and assert yourself calmly with a doctor or midwife regarding your options, showing them that you fully understand your rights, you will usually be given all the support you need to achieve your dream birth. Once a decision has been made and agreed upon with your care providers, you will be given a personalised care plan that is arranged by a senior midwife, and documentation will be written up and put in place behind the scenes to ensure your wishes are followed as closely as possible.

## Your Dream Birth Hierarchy of Needs

What does your dream birth look like? What do you want to achieve on the day? Where do you want to be? How do you see it going in your mind's eye? Every single one of us will desire something different from our experience, and it is your job to work out what you want. After reading through the chapters of this book and attending your antenatal course and birth planning sessions with your partner, you will be ready to put strategies in place. The knowledge and skills you have learned together will help you succeed in achieving the birth of your dreams and support you to reach your true potential.

Sheryl Wynne, an experienced doula and antenatal educator from Simply Natal (**www.simplynatal.co.uk**), specialises in supporting clients who have been through a traumatic birth or postnatal experience. She adapted her 'Healing Birth Hierarchy of Needs' from Maslow's theory of human behaviour. Sheryl says 'We might worry about planning for our dream birth, because it is often seen as black and white—we either get it or we don't! With the birth hierarchy of needs, it's more like a ladder. If we don't get to the top, that's ok, but the higher we can get up the hierarchy, the more empowered our experience will be.'

- **Basic Birth.** The first step on the ladder is to meet your physiological needs: food, water, comfort. At the very least, your birth should include having your physiological needs met at all times. However, many of my clients share that during labour they didn't eat or drink at all, and that labour was long and exhausting, resulting in a very traumatic experience. Don't make this mistake. Nurture yourself throughout the process. If your care provider tells you that you cannot eat or drink in labour—remember you are not in jail. You have the right to do whatever you need in order to sustain your energy.

- **Safe Birth.** The second step is to meet your safety needs: spiritual, mental, emotional. Being supported throughout labour by having your human rights respected by your care providers is essential to having a safe birth experience. You will need to express your wishes and be clear on your spiritual, mental, and emotional needs—ideally in advance so that your wishes can be documented. If during labour you are attended by anyone that makes you feel unsafe, you or your birth partner should request another person to provide you with care.

- **Positive Birth.** The third step supports you to have a positive birth experience, offering love, connection, and oxytocin. As you move up the ladder you can see that in order to achieve a physiological birth, you will definitely require all elements of this step, as you cannot give birth without oxytocin. It is an essential ingredient to the process and is powered by feeling safe and loved. Ensure your birth partner understands the importance of this incredible hormone and protects your oxytocin at all times. They need to fully understand how it is produced and more importantly, what can affect its production.

- **Empowered Birth.** The fourth step is a transformative or empowering birth where you receive support, respect, belief, self-esteem. By taking ownership, and boosting your knowledge of the birthing process, the role of your birth partner, and your rights, you should receive better support and respectful, personalised maternity care. My tips for reaching this level include not letting anyone override your wishes, being consistent, and being clear on your 'why.'

- **Dream Birth.** The fifth step is where you reach your full potential. I want everyone to reach this level; however, if not, my hope is that you get as close as you can. You can climb the ladder and at the very least have an empowered birth experience by remaining in control of your options at all times.

## Your Dream Birth Hierarchy of Needs

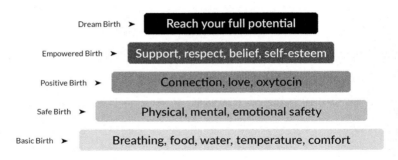

Dream Birth ➤ Reach your full potential

Empowered Birth ➤ Support, respect, belief, self-esteem

Positive Birth ➤ Connection, love, oxytocin

Safe Birth ➤ Physical, mental, emotional safety

Basic Birth ➤ Breathing, food, water, temperature, comfort

The higher up the ladder you go, the more in control you will feel. Even if you don't achieve your dream birth, you can still have an empowering experience. For many this is the chance to heal from a previous birth where, sadly, they didn't even get off the first step of the ladder. I consider most of these steps essential requirements to birth and the early postnatal period. You need to work out what type of birth *you* want to achieve, then figure out how to make it happen. Prepare well and don't accept anything less than the best for your labour. You should be treated with respect at all times and feel well supported.

## Consider Giving Birth at Home

If you are determined to achieve a physiological birth, I recommend you give serious consideration to booking a homebirth. As mammals, we are made to give birth in our own natural habitat, with no external influences. This means your own comfortable home environment, where you feel safe and in control, can facilitate the best level of hormone production possible. Leaving your warm, cosy birth space to go into a foreign and unfamiliar setting, surrounded by strangers, is most likely going to reduce your oxytocin and un-do your hard work. As you know, nothing is ever set in stone, so you can change your mind at any point, acknowledging that if your instincts and physical signs suggest you are not in the right environment, you can transfer to hospital. By having this option on the table, you will be able to spend time discovering if it feels like a good choice for you.

## Packing a Birth Bag

Regardless of where you plan to give birth, it's a good idea to have all the items you want to use during labour in one place. I recommend packing everything into a small bag that can easily be moved from room to room. Show your birth partner where everything is and what each item is for, so that they know how to access these comfort measures and snacks on the day.

Ideas on what to include:

- **Essentials.** Bendy straw, lip balm, eye mask, flannels, homeopathic remedies, aromatherapy oils, music.
- **Snacks.** Honey, jelly, yogurt, banana, chocolate, runners' gel, dried fruit, frozen berries, smoothies, juice shots, ice lollies, coconut water, isotonic drinks.
- **For you.** A clean outfit in case the clothes you are wearing get wet or dirty.
- **For your baby.** A vest, sleepsuit and nappy, and a bag with a few muslin cloths in that you have slept with (see Chapter 1).
- **For your partner.** A change of clothes, toothbrush and toothpaste.
- **For the postnatal period.** I recommend a separate bag with any other items you will need. If you are giving birth in hospital, this bag can be left in the car until after the baby is born; you won't need it during labour. You will find a handy list of recommended items in the free downloads that accompany this book.

Birth Plans **203**

## Find Your 'WHY'

It's important to really nail down your reasons for choosing why you want to give birth physiologically. It's no good planning a homebirth because your friend had one and liked it. You have to really believe in your body and its capabilities. You should fully understand how to let your oxytocin flow and keep it flowing. You must trust your instincts and always come back to your 'why' if a friend, family member or medical professional shows doubt in your plans. You need to prepare your birth partner to fully understand their role and not disturb the process with questions or lack of confidence. Help them identify what established labour looks like, so you don't call the midwife or leave for the hospital too soon, knowing the chance of interventions increases once the clock starts ticking. Know your rights, understand what you can and cannot ask for, and practice saying 'no' to anyone who is trying to persuade you to accept medical support that you do not want.

## Be an Advocate for your Baby

Your baby's birth experience will affect not only you, but also your child as they grow and develop—often in deeper ways than you realise. Being evicted from the womb too soon, being exposed to drugs or antibiotics, or being pulled with instruments can have adverse effects. Whilst sometimes there is a need for medical intervention, most of the time there isn't, making such effects on your baby unnecessary. During my first birth, I was told I had to have antibiotics during labour as I had been diagnosed with Group B strep, a common bacteria found in the vagina that can lead to infection in a small percentage of babies. The antibiotics had a profound effect on my son—on his skin, his sleep, and his digestive system—that still impacts him in adulthood. If I had researched Group B strep more thoroughly and understood the risks and alternatives (including avoiding vaginal examinations) I would never have chosen to accept them. I declined all recommendations for my subsequent 3 children.

## Fran's Story

*Fran had given birth to her daughter Zoe in hospital after a long induction. Eventually, after prolonged pushing, she was moved to theatre and Zoe was born with the use of metal forceps. In the days following the birth, Fran noticed that Zoe wasn't holding her head correctly and was crying all the time. Realising she was uncomfortable; she called the midwife for support and was booked into see the doctor. Zoe was diagnosed with Torticollis, where the nerves in her neck were compressed, and the muscles were stiff. She struggled to turn her head without pain. Fran was able to take Zoe to a local cranial osteopath and had a series of gentle treatments that helped ease the problem. When Fran was pregnant again, she had ensured everyone was aware that an instrumental birth using forceps or ventouse was a hard boundary for her, and she would not be accepting another induction.*

## Writing Your Birth Plan

The last few years have seen birth plans become more widely accepted by medical professionals, and there are now some amazing resources online with novel ideas about how to document your preferences, including using pictures and diagrams. I personally believe that images can be confusing to your care providers, and I don't think they are the best way to convey your preferences. Similarly, remember that midwives and doctors are busy and won't have time to read through too much detail. By identifying what you feel are the most important elements, you will be able to write clear and direct points that convey your wishes, and not spend time writing pages of information that will be overlooked. It is also important that the instructions within the birth plan are relevant to the location you are giving birth in, to ensure they relate specifically to the care providers in that environment. There is no need to include the elements you want your partner to take care of, such as keeping lights off, playing relaxing music, giving you remedies, feeding you snacks and drinks, and using props like peanut balls. Prepare your birth partner well so that they understand what every point on the plan correlates to, and what your boundaries are regarding each one; this will help them if they find themselves in a situation where they need to advocate for you. I also find a birth plan particularly useful when a woman I am supporting has stated a preference, but the midwife overlooks this preference or wants her to reconsider. For example: Let's say that on your birth plan you have indicated you would like to leave the umbilical cord to finish pulsating. Then, early in the post-natal period, when you are both happily gazing at the baby, you notice the midwife getting ready to clamp the cord. At this point, your birth partner can remind them of your choice, and your midwife will know this is a decision you have made in advance of birth that is not being influenced by the person supporting you. This is particularly important if the midwife or doctor is refusing to accept any verbal instructions from your partner, and only wants to hear your preferences directly from you. A written birth plan can be very useful in this common scenario.

## Birth Plan Samples

Once you are ready to start writing your birth plan and feel confident in your knowledge about all your options, you can begin by considering the points that you really want to get across to the person providing you with care. Be really clear and concise, ensuring you identify any hard boundaries that are important. Here are three birth plan examples that fall within the guidelines of physiological birth. You can write one similar or different to these; just keep them simple. You can also write separate plans for B and C to support you in the event that you need them—but keep them tucked away in your birth bag.

## Sample Plan 1

### Preferences

**Yes, Please**

- Use the pool if it is available
- Gas and air will be considered
- Optimal cord clamping
- Immediate skin-to-skin contact

**No, Thanks**

- Talking, especially during a contraction
- Electronic Fetal Monitor
- Vaginal examinations

## Sample Plan 2

- I am hypnobirthing.
- I would like to use the birth pool if it's available.
- I would like to avoid vaginal examinations.
- Please do not offer me pain relief. I am aware of what is available and will ask for some if required.
- I do not want to push until I feel the urge.
- I would like to leave the umbilical cord to stop pulsating, and allow the placenta to come away on its own without the use of an oxytocin injection.
- I would like immediate skin to skin contact for at least an hour after the baby is born to establish bonding and feeding. Please do not put a hat on the baby.
- If medical management becomes necessary, I will decline any offer of an induction and would like to have a C-section.

**Sample Plan 3**

I am planning a physiological birth with no interventions

I am hypnobirthing

I would like to have a water birth

**I consent to...**

- Physical checks like pulse and blood pressure
- Listening to the baby's heart rate with a doppler
- Vitamin K

**I do not consent to...**

- Vaginal examinations
- Cervical sweeps
- Episiotomy
- Cutting the umbilical cord before it is white, empty, and finished pulsating

I do not want to feel any pressure to give birth in a set time frame, and I would prefer to avoid any analytical discussions about my labour.

I have a safety word in place, which will enable me to vocalise freely.

If I decide to use any birth management methods, I know what is available and will use my safety word in order to discuss what I would like to do next.

My partner and my doula will advocate for me. I hope that you will respect their voices, as they fully understand my wishes. I give them full permission to speak on my behalf if necessary.

If at any point a decision needs to be made, I would appreciate if you shared with us all risks and benefits regarding your recommendations. We would then like some privacy to consider these.

# Summary

. . . . . . .

- **Understand your options.** Looking at all the options and choices you have available to you locally, and knowing what information you may still need to learn and understand, can help you in preparation for your birth. Go through the birth plan checklist during your first birth planning session and see if there are any gaps in your knowledge. There are many decisions you may be expected to make either in advance of the birth or on the day. By doing your research, you and your birth partner will feel well prepared for all eventualities and be able to make informed decisions if the need arises.

- **Write your birth plan.** When looking at the examples in this chapter, you should get a really good idea about how to write an easy-to-read list of your preferences. Don't write an essay, or a copious amount of information that is hard to read and understand by the person caring for you, who is probably extremely busy and has other women to care for at the same time. Take great care to make your points clear and concise and keep to one side of A4 paper or less if possible. You can write a separate Plan B and C if that helps you to feel well prepared, but put them in your bag and only bring them to your care provider if it becomes necessary.

- **Recognise the value of a birth plan for your partner.** It is not uncommon for a care provider to override your birth partner and only listen to you regarding decisions that may need to be made. I have heard of clients being taken aside and asked if they were in an abusive relationship. The midwife or doctor did not want to accept the word of the partner over the woman, so it's a good idea to have a way of communicating your wishes to your care provider clearly without the need for clarification if you are unable to speak at any given time.

# CHAPTER 8
## *Final Preparations*

*Impatience leads to intervention.*

These five key principles—understanding your hormones, trusting your instincts, preparing your birth partner, knowing your rights, and believing in your body—are essential to planning and achieving a physiological birth. This final chapter will consolidate the information shared with you consistently throughout the book and give you some final tips about taking ownership of your birth experience. Then, if you attend a consultation with your care provider, and an intervention is recommended, you will understand what is being asked of you and be able to have an informed conversation. I want to make sure that your birth won't be sabotaged because of an inaccurate comment, or that a perceived risk relayed to you leads you to believe an intervention is essential when it isn't. Most recommendations made to pregnant women about their care are not evidence based but merely the opinion of the care provider. Anyone who wants to give birth without medical management should know there is a lot to be learned about nature's design, and a lot to be gained from deeply trusting your body and your baby. The experience of physiological childbirth and the intensity it can bring is not for everyone, but if it is for *you*, then you deserve full support from anyone providing you with care, so that you are treated respectfully, your wishes are met, and your experience kept safe and not disrupted or ruined by the careless disregard of others. I also want you to feel confident in knowing why, for the vast majority of women, it's best to avoid having your baby in a main hospital obstetric unit, as it can put you both at greater risk. The deep level of mistrust and impatience many doctors have regarding the birth process is leading to interventions on an epic scale. Women are left broken, and they and their babies are being pumped with drugs and antibiotics that have a huge effect on their lives postnatally. It is vital to ensure that you are well prepared and remain in control of all decisions about your birth. We need to get back to the days when you could just turn up to your midwife appointment for a chat and a wellbeing check, then call the midwife out to you at home when the time comes, with no fuss or concerns, whilst you gently birth your baby.

## Making Decisions

If you know all your options, you will feel well prepared to make decisions at any stage, especially if your labour has elements to it that you did not expect. You can make informed decisions if things develop, so that you are able to say 'yes' to what you want, but you are also confident and capable of saying 'no' to what you don't! It's about giving birth to your baby in a way that meets your needs, and not the needs and timing of your care providers. The birth partner's role is equally important here, so they can successfully advocate for you and support you to achieve as much of the birth you are planning as possible. Your birth support team needs to know what you want, what they can do to help you, and fundamentally they need to know 'why.' If your birth partner doesn't get the 'why,' they can drop their support in favour of listening to the opinion of a medical professional who is overriding you. This is where the deepest trauma can occur, leaving you feeling betrayed by your birth partner, so help them understand the 'why' for whatever you are choosing.

## Extra Tests and Checks

The more appointments, extra scans, and additional checks you attend, the more you will be exposing yourself to care provider fear. In the UK, for example, if your midwife recommends you attend the antenatal clinic for further tests, it is automatically assumed you will see the doctor. If you do not want to be exposed to conversations regarding your care, you can decline. If you choose to go, remember you do not have to be held back by other people's fear and doubt in your abilities. It can be incredibly upsetting and disempowering if during an appointment you are met with comments from a doctor or midwife that belittle your knowledge, especially if you have taken time to investigate your options thoroughly. Their beliefs should not be affecting choices and decisions that come from a place of instinct. In my experience, the stumbling block is usually the need to please and be liked. You may have been told as a child to be obedient and well behaved, to smile and not question authority. This is often referred to as 'good girl' syndrome, and we internalise these messages from a young age. Understandably, no one wants to be the difficult one, the complainer, the person who seems ungrateful or annoying. What's important is to remember you are not being difficult. You simply want to own your birth experience and make it the best it can be— and you are just better informed than most people! So smile and be kind, but also be firm and clear and consistent about your ability to give birth in the way you are planning, and even if doubts or fears arise, you can quickly let them go, always bringing your thoughts back to the confidence you have in your body and baby.

## Emma's Story

*Emma's first baby was over 4 kg at birth, so considered big. When she became pregnant with her second child it was flagged as a concern, and she was automatically offered a glucose tolerance test (GTT) to check for gestational diabetes. Emma wanted to decline the test, as she had been keeping a close eye on her food intake and knew that for anyone who is eating a healthy diet, the test results can give a false positive. She also didn't want an induction of labour at 39 weeks which she knew her doctor would push for if the GTT showed raised glucose levels. The midwives strongly encouraged her to be tested, making her feel difficult and irresponsible for declining. After lots of research, instead of rejecting the test completely, Emma agreed to use a continuous glucose monitor to pacify them. Her readings were well within the normal range, but when she had two results that were slightly above the cut-off point, Emma was labelled as having gestational diabetes anyway. We spent a lot of time together discussing this misdiagnosis and how to avoid it affecting her decision to give birth physiologically. We knew the two readings that triggered the positive result could easily have been slightly above normal due to lack of sleep and feeling stressed. As all of her other readings were low and well within the normal range, she was confident that there was nothing to be concerned about for either her or the baby. Despite the pressure and constant scare tactics around the risks of remaining pregnant, Emma found the courage to decline all further testing and the offer of induction. She went on to achieve a beautiful physiological birth to another 'big' baby who was born quickly and easily.*

## Ticking Clock

Impatience already exists within the maternity system, so it's important not to add fuel to the fire and buy into the idea that the clock is ticking regarding the end of your pregnancy.

I know it's hard when you are really looking forward to meeting your baby (and maybe are weary of being pregnant!) but let's look at some of the benefits of giving birth physiologically. These include the baby's lungs being fully mature; microbes being primed and ready to start building a healthy immune system; and hormones being released to provide you both with the ability to birth quickly, bond easily, and feed efficiently. If all of these are preparing your baby for the outside world, then why rush the process before the baby is lined up and ready? The idea of a ticking clock always makes me think of a bomb waiting to go off—but you are not a bomb. You are a pregnant woman with a developing baby inside you, who will soon enough trigger those hormones, given their own time. The ticking clock is real for medical professionals, however, and once labour is underway, you may feel pressure to give birth reasonably quickly. Local hospital guidelines typically suggest for example, that after your waters break you will be 'allowed' up to 24 hours before the on-duty doctor will want to begin the induction process. If you have a vaginal examination, it will be expected that your cervix dilate by one centimetre every two hours, and once you begin pushing, they will want your baby to be born within an hour and a half before they intervene. Remember that guidelines are only relevant to you if you want them to be. You can say 'yes' or 'no' to each and every one. Avoiding these pressures and time constraints is not easy, but if physiological birth is important to you, consider the following.

- Be really aware of your baby's regular activities. What are the patterns that your baby makes each day? What is normal for them? By having a clear understanding of their regular day-to-day movements within the womb, your instincts will tell you if your baby is doing well and your pregnancy can continue despite offers or recommendations of induction. You can back this up with regular appointments to listen to the baby's heartbeat, check your blood pressure, and/or attend scans at the hospital to check amniotic fluid levels.

- It is important to avoid seeking care too early in labour. If everything is going well, remain at home, and don't leave for the hospital or invite a midwife to your homebirth until you are confident you are in established labour. To be clear, this involves consistent contractions that are coming regularly, lasting around the same length of time (approximately one minute) and forming a pattern. If you are having short and long contractions that stop or start when you change position, or if a disturbance occurs that disrupts the pattern, then labour is not established. A clear sign that you are advancing is when, after each contraction subsides, you need to take a moment to recover, are not interested in external distractions, and don't want to talk.

- Once in labour, decline vaginal examinations. They are offered upon arrival and are then expected to be performed every 4 hours. You may be put under pressure to accept one with the classic line, 'how will we know if you are in labour if we don't check your cervix?' If no examination is done, the clock cannot begin ticking as they have no line in the sand to work from.

- Avoid any directed pushing or anything you might describe as a feeling or sensation to push. If your body is not giving you an overwhelming urge that you couldn't stop if you tried, then your body and your baby are not quite ready. When the body takes over and the baby is aligned, you will begin pushing without needing to ask yourself if you are pushing. It will be obvious to all around you, and your body will be doing it instinctively. I describe this as being the same as feeling like you need a poo versus pooing, or the difference between feeling nauseous and actually vomiting.

## Overcoming Impatience

When labour does begin, never ever chase it! If you try to bring on or speed up the birthing process, you can meddle and change outcomes—typically for the worse, not the better. Some examples include cervical sweeps, where I have seen longer more drawn out labours, or—in some cases—labour moves too fast and is overwhelming, leaving you feeling traumatised; sitting on a birth ball and rocking around in an attempt to get things moving prematurely, which can exhaust you and deplete your energy too early; or using remedies to stimulate contractions before the baby is in alignment, leading to a long and difficult labour. The success of achieving a physiological birth relies upon all five principles outlined in this book, but in addition, overcoming impatience is crucial. In order to remind yourself of this anytime you are feeling a little restless whilst waiting for your baby to be born, here are two mantras you can say repeatedly to yourself:

*My baby will come when they are ready.*
*When my body is in charge, very little will go wrong.*

No matter where you are in your pregnancy journey, you may need to repeat these mantras many times so that they sink deep into your subconscious mind. Becoming aware of your own personality traits will help you overcome some levels of impatience in advance of birth. If, for example, you like a lot of control in your life, then you might find it difficult to relax and wait for your baby to come in their own time. It helps to let go of relying on your due date (see Chapter 6) because it's more likely you will give birth in the week following. The more you focus on a certain date, the longer each day beyond that date can feel, leaving you vulnerable and more likely to accept any suggested interventions you hear from your care provider. If you have a doula, birth keeper or independent midwife providing you with care and support in pregnancy, there is less chance you will feel pressured to give birth before your baby is ready, but if not, you may begin to feel that you are running out of time with each day that passes.

## Limiting Beliefs

A limitless birth is about ensuring that your body can birth physiologically and not be held back by beliefs that prevent you from reaching your true potential. Limiting beliefs live deep down in your subconscious mind and can really hold you back in life. Do you ever think to yourself 'I can't do it,' 'I'm not good enough,' or 'I have a low pain threshold'? These classic limiting beliefs do not serve you. Giving birth is often perceived as something to tolerate, a means to an end. I have no doubt that for many it is that way. But it doesn't have to be; it can be beautiful, spiritual, and sensual. It can be anything you put your mind to, because you have the power to change the thoughts in your mind to match your ideas, helping you to give birth without limits and thereby succeed in achieving your dream birth.

Limiting beliefs manifest in stories that start with:

- I am not allowed to... (give birth at home)
- I had to have... (an induction)
- I can't have... (a water birth)
- They booked me in for an ... (abdominal birth)

If you use a sentence that starts with one of these examples, you are transforming a recommendation made to you into a story that prevents you from exploring your options further. A doctor or midwife cannot tell you how you can give birth, because they don't have the right to decide for you. Only you do! If anyone providing care is not supportive of your decisions, you may have to switch them for someone who is.

If, however, you were to have a conversation about your care that was realistic, truthful, inclusive, supportive, and balanced, you might decide to agree with any recommendations made, but your telling of the story would be different and more like:

- I decided against a homebirth because it no longer felt like a safe place for my baby to be born...
- I chose an induction in the end because after weighing up the pros and cons, we felt it was the right decision at the time...
- I realised that having a waterbirth was no longer an option for me as I wanted to give birth on labour ward and there was no pool...
- We felt that an abdominal birth was the right decision for us after long discussions with the doctor about the circumstances we found ourselves in...

Then, you have made well informed decisions. But to not know why you are not allowed, or to agree to something that you didn't want without good reason, might lead to disappointment.

## Getting Rid of Limiting Beliefs

When thinking about and planning your physiological birth experience, your focus should be on cultivating a deep level of trust in your body to continue what it started, and on protecting yourself from any negative thoughts that could sabotage your plans and distract you from your instincts. Your job is to eliminate self-doubt and step into your power.

Ways to do this might include:
- Identifying what your limiting beliefs are and recognising that they are just beliefs

- Challenging the beliefs that you have, and doing your research to ensure you know the supporting facts
- Adopting a new belief and then starting to focus on what you want
- Wrapping yourself and your baby up in an invisible bubble of protection, to avoid absorbing other people's unsupportive words.

This can take time for many people, so start as early as possible. You can then begin to let go of the limiting beliefs you have. It's not always easy, and you may find the old habits kicking in, and these negative thoughts popping back up at times, so be kind to yourself. A trick I recommend to my clients if they feel negative thoughts arising is to immediately begin counting backwards from 10 – 1. This works well to get rid of the thought, feeling, or doubt, helping you to move past it.

## Minerals and Hydration

It's incredibly beneficial for you to understand how mineral and hydration levels can affect the health and well-being of both you and your baby, and the influence it will have on your postnatal journey. By learning more, you can ensure your body is in tip-top condition to support you to achieve a physiological birth (or any birth for that matter). First, it's important to remember we aren't all perfect, and we need balance in our lives, so please don't dwell on what you have or haven't eaten so far but remind yourself that it's never too late to make changes. Any adaptations you make moving forward will reward you by improving your health and wellness for your future. Learning about minerals and understanding the role they play will support the changes your body is experiencing and improve your overall physical abilities and general well being. Minerals such as magnesium, potassium, choline, calcium, zinc, and sodium are all vital to everyone's health, but are even more important to you, with the demands that pregnancy and breast feeding will have on your body. They not only conduct energy, but create it, and are critical for the body to function. Deficiencies have been associated with conditions such as pre-eclampsia, hypertension, oedema (swelling), gestational diabetes, premature labour, abruption of the placenta and more. Low levels of magnesium and potassium for example are associated with higher fasting blood glucose levels. By addressing these deficiencies, you can prevent or control some of the conditions listed above. The best way to increase minerals in your diet is to eat foods such as nuts and seeds, beans and lentils, dark leafy greens and cruciferous vegetables, fish, eggs, mushrooms, whole grains, dairy, beef and lamb, avocados, tofu, bananas, dark chocolate, cheese and dried fruits. Be sure to prioritise high quality meats, eggs, and dairy products to support your body's changes and the growth of you and your baby. If your minerals come from whole foods rather than from supplementation, your body can then use these minerals to replenish and balance electrolytes, which are as important to you as proteins, fats, carbohydrates and vitamins. Electrolytes are essential for energy, adrenal health, and fluid balance, helping to prevent common pregnancy symptoms like headaches and cramps. As your pregnancy develops, your blood volume increases, and your body needs to remain well hydrated. This is important for circulation, absorption of nutrients and digestion. You can increase your fluid levels by eating salads and fruits with a high-water content. Also prioritise fluids that naturally contain minerals such as coconut water which is high in potassium, or herbal teas (choose ones that are safe to drink in pregnancy) as well as water.

## Not Everyone Likes Calm and Relaxation

I want to acknowledge that staying calm and relaxed isn't for everyone. I appreciate that some of you will prefer giving birth in a busy environment, having friends and family around you, hearing lots of chatter, and keeping the room bright and cheerful. Some of my clients simply don't like passive relaxation techniques and prefer to use alternative birth management methods that are more stimulating. Two methods I recommend are stress balls or a comb. Both are held in the hands, and work on the gate control theory, where you give the brain something to focus on and divert your attention from the sensation of the contraction, producing endorphins at the same time. If energy is present due to the arrival of adrenaline, this technique can help you make the most of that extra energy, channelling it in a different way.

- **Stress Balls.** These should be medium or soft resistance, not hard like tennis balls, and can be coloured for extra visual focus. You can squeeze and release the stress balls, finding a rhythm that suits you best. You might like to tap the balls together as your sensations intensify. You can also make sounds as you bring the balls together in a repetitive way. You could choose to use other items that provide sensory stimulation like amethyst rocks, squeeze toys, balls with bells or lights, play dough, or clay.

- **Comb.** You can use any comb that fits in the palm of your hand; however, there are combs that are perfectly designed for labour, like the Wave Comb. When you feel a contraction, you push the bristles into the palm of your hand, helping you to experience an alternative sensation to focus on. This also gives you the added bonus of hitting an acupressure point, which releases energy.

## Doubts: Part of the Survival Mechanism

In advance of labour, and during, you are highly likely to feel moments of uncertainty, both in yourself and about the decisions you are making. This is physiologically normal and related to the negative bias we have built into us for survival. Ride any waves of doubt you feel and embrace them; you will come out the other side. Sometimes you might forget to breathe or make loud sounds and behave in a way that you didn't expect. Don't beat yourself up afterwards if you say negative words or acted in a less-than-serene way, particularly if this wasn't how you imagined yourself behaving. Just ensure that you have all the tools you need nearby to get back on track. Have a safety word in place so you can vocalise as much as you want and trust that your birth partner will know you are not looking to be rescued. Warn them in advance that if you say you are struggling, or that you can't do it, they should simply remind you how amazing you are, and give you a gentle smile or a hug. Words of affirmation can really help in this situation, so prepare your partner with short sentences that will encourage you to keep believing in yourself. I once heard a story of a man who wanted to run 100 miles but couldn't get past 35 miles. He hired a coach who shared only one tip: to keep saying to himself 'I never get tired.' The next day he completed 100 miles, and to everyone he met along the way, he repeated his mantra by telling them he never gets tired. It worked like magic.

### Exposure to Antibiotics

With the rise in fear-based practice, more and more babies being born in hospital are exposed to antibiotics in the early postnatal period. Paediatricians act on a just-in-case basis, with concerns that your baby 'might' develop an infection, particularly if there are any risk factors, such as your waters breaking in advance of labour. If the baby is born in a facility where there is no paediatric cover, for example, home or an MLU, the same concerns do not apply. It's merely a 'not on my watch' scenario, where doctors will look for any possible reason to suspect an issue. Whilst I am sure you are delighted to know that all paediatricians want to keep your baby safe, the decision to offer antibiotics 'just in case' they develop an infection, should not be left to them. I am not talking about life-saving treatments here, with a confirmed deadly infection or a serious life-threatening condition. I am talking about the overuse of antibiotics which could put your baby at more harm in the future, if your child genuinely needs antibiotics and has become resistant. You can absolutely overrule a doctor if they want to give your baby antibiotics without your permission, particularly if the pros do not outweigh the cons. You have parental rights that make you responsible for your child, and a doctor cannot overrule you unless there is a life-threatening situation. Asking for evidence-based information and having respectful discussion about your reasoning is essential. Antibiotics affect the gut dramatically, causing an imbalance in the microbiome before it has even had a chance to develop. This can contribute to long term health conditions such as: Eczema, Acne, Asthma, Allergies, Diabetes, Coeliac, IBS, mental health issues, chronic fatigue, Parkinson's disease, MS and other immune system diseases. In the early days of a baby's life, the more common results of such an imbalance are thrush, skin issues, and sleep problems. In addition, you may be required to stay in hospital for as many as 7 days or longer, where your baby will be given intravenous antibiotics every 12 hours, which no one explains to you at the time.

If your baby does receive antibiotics, either because you were given them during an abdominal birth or because they became essential in the early postnatal period, then do your best to help re-colonise their gut with your own bacteria as quickly as possible, with lots of skin-to-skin time and by feeding them colostrum. I recommend that you have three or four blankets or muslin cloths that you have slept with during pregnancy available in your birth bag (see Chapter 1). You can also purchase a high-quality probiotic—both a paediatric one suitable for newborns and an extra strength one for you. If you are curious to find out more about how important the microbiome is to a newborn baby, watch the amazing film "Microbirth" made by Toni Harman and Alex Wakeford. Released in 2014, this incredible documentary investigates the latest scientific research on the microscopic events happening during childbirth. These events can have serious implications for the lifelong health of children.

## Wild Pregnancy and Freebirth

Wild pregnancy, where a woman declines any antenatal care, and freebirth, where she chooses to give birth at home without a midwife present, is a legal right here in the UK and many other countries around the world. The two are very different, and not mutually exclusive, so whilst one woman might decline scans but happily give birth in hospital, another might choose to accept all antenatal care but give birth alone. Others will take the decision to decline all antenatal appointments and have a freebirth. Since 2020 and the start of the Covid 19 pandemic, there has been a significant rise in women declining care, since so many were let down by the withdrawal of both partner support during antenatal appointments and homebirth services in their area. Women began to feel confident in continuing their plans to give birth at home despite knowing that medical support had been withdrawn. Facebook groups like **Homebirth Support Group UK**, led by Samantha Gadsden, saw membership numbers escalate with many signing up to attend her freebirth course during this time in preparation for giving birth without assistance. Stories began to flood in from women who had their babies with just their partner and sometimes a family member, friend, or doula present. So many beautiful tales of undisturbed birth from women who went to great lengths to learn about and prepare for their physiological birth. These stories inspired others to freebirth and/or decline antenatal appointments, checks, or scans. If you are considering the idea of declining some or all antenatal care including having a freebirth, I recommend you sign up to Sam's course (link in the resource section), read books like *Unassisted Childbirth* by Laura Shanley, and listen to my podcast with guest Leonie Rainbird-Savin, who shared her 3 very different stories of freebirth. If you decide you are interested in giving birth unassisted, there is much to learn, so do your research and enter into the experience feeling well prepared.

## Preparation for Birth

As you know, this book is not a complete antenatal course, and a lot of the details within assume that you understand key elements of antenatal education. When choosing a course to attend with your partner, pick wisely, as courses vary. I recommend attending a course with an experienced birth professional who really understands physiological birth and can see that you cement your knowledge with a balanced viewpoint. Many course providers have no experience in attending births other than their own, so they can only share routine information with you. If you want to deepen your knowledge about all aspects of birth and attend a course that offers your birth partner a greater level of awareness and understanding of their role in supporting you, consider signing up for one of my courses **www.birthability.co.uk** (see links at the back of the book). I can personally help you and your birth partner build on the information that you need to know, in preparation for achieving your dream birth.

## What's Your Backup Plan?

There is no harm in having a Plan B or C. Despite all the chat about mindset and limiting beliefs, it's impossible to 100% guarantee that your birth will go the way you are planning. If you find yourself in a situation where it's obvious you will need interventions, or you yourself decide you want to ask for extra support, then do so with confidence and always remain in control. Choosing to accept an induction or abdominal birth for really valid reasons, asking for a vaginal examination because you want to make a new plan, or deciding to get out of the pool and have an epidural are all brilliant ways to move forward when you know it's what you want. Remember to use your safety word to ensure your partner is aware that you are not just vocalising but are definite that you want to change course. If you prefer, you can write a birth plan for Plans B and C if it helps you to feel organised and well prepared; just keep them in your bag until needed. If things do deviate from your Plan A, that doesn't mean you've given up control; you've just made new decisions that come from a place of knowledge and even more power, knowing those are your decisions to make.

## Step into Your Power

It's time to step into your power and be the hero of your birth story. Babies are not delivered in a box like a gift with a bow; they are born, and you are the one giving birth to them. It's you that experiences the magic of your changing body making space for your growing baby, you that feels them moving inside you, you that will feel the powerful sensations that will bring them into the world to meet you—and all this happens without you ever needing to think or do anything.

So believe in the rest of the story, and allow your birth experience to flow. You are hard wired to do this. There are no clocks ticking—they are all imaginary—so if you can just lean into the journey and trust the process, you will have a pretty special time.

*You've always had the power, my dear—*
*you just had to learn it for yourself.*

–Glinda the Good Witch

# Resources

To make it easier for you to access information from these websites, I have included a list of all the clickable links on my website. From there, you will also be able to access the free downloads that accompany this book: **bit.ly/theartofgivingbirth.**

Antenatal Education

Sallyann Beresford   **birthability.co.uk**

Megan Rossiter   **birth-ed.co.uk**

Sheryl Wynne   **simplynatal.co.uk**

Emma Armstrong   **thenakeddoula.me**

Carmen Cardoso   **linktr.ee/Carmenthebirthcoach**

Births of Multiples

Twins Trust   **twinstrust.org**

Birth Partners (my book)

Labour of Love: The Ultimate Guide
to Being a Birth Partner   **bit.ly/Labouroflove**

Birth Support
>  Doula UK   **doula.org.uk**
>  Independent Midwives UK   **imuk.org.uk**

Birth Trauma
>  Birth Trauma Association
>  **birthtraumaassociation.org.uk**

Breastfeeding Support
>  Breastfeeding Support   **breastfeeding.support**
>  Kelly Mom   **kellymom.com**
>  Association for Breastfeeding Mothers   **abm.me.uk**
>  La Leche League   **laleche.org.uk**

Caesarean Birth
>  Caesarean Birth   **caesarean.org.uk**

Diet and Nutrition
>  Lily Nichols   **lilynicholsrdn.com**
>  The Brewers Diet   **drbrewerpregnancydiet.com**

Evidence-Based Resources

    Mothers and Babies Reducing Risks through Audits
        (MBRRACE-UK)   **npeu.ox.ac.uk/mbrrace-uk**

    Midwife Thinking   **midwifethinking.com**

    Evidence Based Birth   **evidencebasedbirth.com**

    Sara Wickham   **sarawickham.com**

    Sarah Buckley   **sarahbuckley.com**

Freebirth

    Samantha Gadsden   **caerphillydoula.co.uk**

Guidelines

    Royal College of Obstetricians and
        Gynaecologists   **rcog.org.uk**

    National Institute for Health and Care Excellence
        (NICE)   **nice.org.uk**

    Royal College of Midwives (RCM)   **rcm.org.uk**

    Royal College of Anaesthetists (RCoA)   **rcoa.ac.uk**

    Royal College of Paediatrics and Child Health
        (RCPCH)   **rcpch.ac.uk**

    Cochrane (Summaries of health evidence)
        **cochrane.org**

## Miscarriage and Stillbirth
Stillbirth and Neonatal Death Charity (Sands)
**sands.org.uk**
Lullaby Trust   **lullabytrust.org.uk**
Tommy's   **tommys.org**
Beyond Bea   **beyondbea.co.uk**

## Optimal Cord Clamping
Wait for White Campaign   **waitforwhite.com**
Ticc Tocc Campaign   **drgreen.com**
Lotus Birth   **babyprepping.com**

## Placenta Encapsulation
Placenta Remedies Network (PRN)
**placentaremediesnetwork.org**

## Podcasts
The Ultimate Birth Partner
Birthing Instincts
The Midwives Cauldron
Birth Ed
The Better Birth

## Pre-and Postnatal Depression
PaNDAS (PND Awareness and Support)
**pandasfoundation.org.uk**

Pregnancy

    Pregnancy Sickness Support
       **pregnancysicknesssupport.org.uk**
    Tell Me a Good Birth Story
       **tellmeagoodbirthstory.com**
    Spinning Babies    **spinningbabies.com**
    Pelvic Partnership (Pelvic Girdle Pain)
       **pelvicpartnership.org.uk**
    Pre-Eclampsia    **preeclampsia.org**
    Breech Birthing    **breechbirthing.com**
    Gloria Lemay    **wisewomanwayofbirth.com**
    Biomechanics    **optimalbirth.co.uk**

Reduced Fetal Movement
    Kicks Count    **kickscount.org.uk**

Support for Women's Rights in Childbirth
    Association for Improvement in Maternity Services
       (AIMS)    **aims.org.uk**
    Birthrights    **birthrights.org.uk**
    National Maternity Voices (NMV) / Maternity Voices
       Partnership (MVP)    **nationalmaternityvoices.org.uk**
    White Ribbon Alliance    **whiteribbonalliance.org**
    Maternity Action    **maternityaction.org.uk**

# Acknowledgments

Writing this book has been an absolute pleasure, giving me the ability to pour my heart and soul into my favourite topic. This was a very different journey to last time, without both lockdowns giving me all the hours in the day I needed to write and edit with no other commitments. Instead, the world kept spinning, with clients giving birth and classes being taught in addition to the writing. Needless to say the end result is amazing and I am so pleased and proud of this incredible resource for women who want to give birth physiologically. I am also extremely grateful to everyone who kindly supported me throughout the process, in particular:

**To Tim**, my very patient and loving husband, who is always encouraging of my writing despite the many tasks at home that never get done. Thank you for choosing me and supporting me in achieving my dreams.

**To Fiona Gordon**, who is a great inspiration to me and a wonderful advocate of my work. I was so thrilled that you offered to help edit the book, as your knowledge and experience has given you the ability to fully understand the concepts I was trying to convey. I am so lucky to have you and your unwavering support in my life. Thank you for always being there for me—you are a very special friend.

**To Emma Winspear**, who patiently read every word and chapter, giving suggestions and ideas to help develop the concept of my 5 key principles. I was incredibly honoured to witness you stepping into your power and owning your experience with your beautiful physiological birth. You helped shape this book into a really useful tool for other women to achieve the same. Thank you so much for your help and for becoming my friend.

**To my four wonderful children, Joe, Lauren, Caitlin, and Darcy**, who continue to be my inspiration for writing books about childbirth. I want to ensure that you all have the ability to experience your dream births at some stage in the future.

**To Sarah Montagu.** Your incredible skills as a midwife gave me the chance to step into my own power and birth in the way I wanted. You sat quietly and held space for me each time and I couldn't be more grateful for your skill at supporting my physiological philosophies.

**To Michel Odent and Liliana Lammers**. I learned so much from you both about physiological birth, and I still implement the tips and tools you shared with me on the doula course I attended all those years ago. Thank you for your contributions to the doula community.

**To the Physiological Birth Club**, including Kemi Johnson, Carmen Rocha, James Bourton, Milly Morris, Leonie Rainbird-Savin, Daisy Dinwoodie, Jenna Brough, Michelle Quashie, Alex Burner and Catherine Cooper to name a few. I have really found my tribe with you all and I truly appreciate the support you offer to me on a regular basis.

**To all the women and their partners** who have invited me to be a part of their birth journeys. Every single one has had an impact on my life, and I feel privileged and grateful to you all.

**To everyone who has given me permission** to use their words in this book—you know who you are.

**And finally to Tessa Avila**. Thank you so much as always for bringing my books to life. Your calm, quiet wisdom and attention to detail makes the process of writing seamless. I am incredibly lucky to have access to your unwavering support and numerous talents, enabling me to share my words with the world. Our friendship means so much, and I am happy to have had you alongside me on this journey once again with your deep knowledge and experience as a mother, editor, and designer.

# Index